TRAIN YOUR MENTAL TOUGHNESS

Build an Unbeatable Mindset By Developing Self Discipline, Resilience and Grit

STEVEN STORM

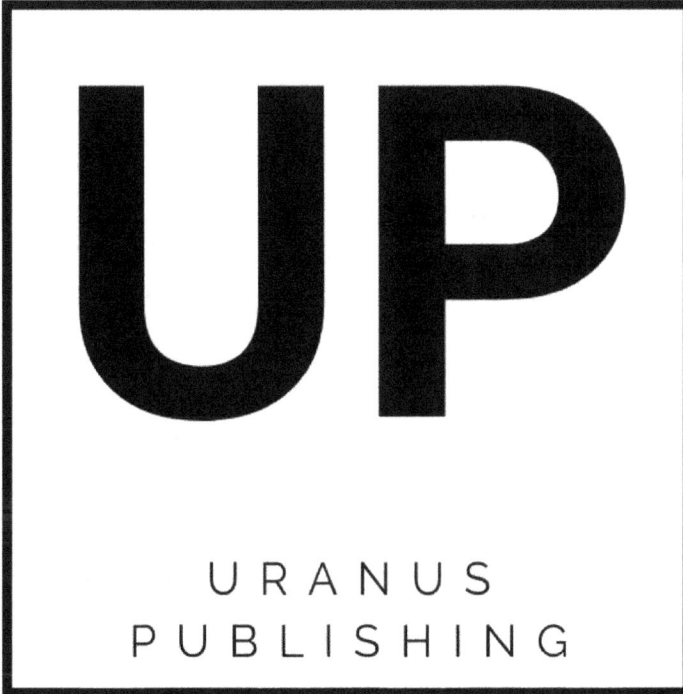

UP

URANUS
PUBLISHING

Paperback ISBN : 978-1-915218-04-9

TABLE OF CONTENTS

INTRODUCTION

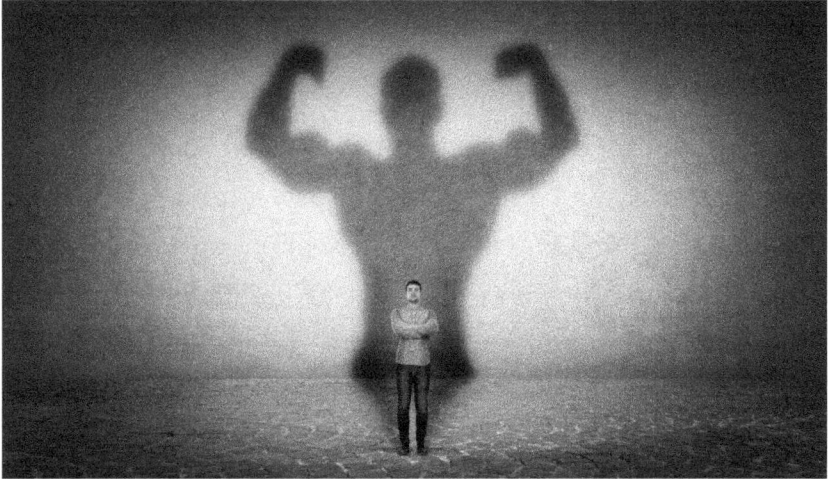

Individuals competing for pure pleasure, leisure, and innocent recreation are uncommon in today's environment. It is also uncommon to hear the remark "it doesn't matter whether we win or lose" — a philosophy that is becoming increasingly out of date.

The world we live in now appears to be more preoccupied with achievement and the desire and drive to "win." Perhaps the concept of being the best, the most strong, or the most intelligent is enticing and encapsulates our desire for achievement. In practically every endeavor that humanity undertakes, there is a desire to be at the top or, at the very least, to continuously improve. In this book, we will explore some thought-provoking topics and answer the following questions: What distinguishes an athlete who thrives on elite competition from one who crumbles under pressure? Why are some athletes able to achieve in the face of hardship while others are unable? Why can some athletes reject and overlook unfavorable competition effects, but others allow them to affect and degrade their competitive performance? What enables athletes to bounce back after defeat and personal failure? Many people believe that the answers to these concerns can be found in the successful development, execution, and ongoing upkeep of mental toughness. Today, top athletes understand that success entails more than simply technique and adds a new dimension known as the "psychology of winning." This involves various mental ingredients such as context-specific mental skills found in tailor-made mental toughness programs.

Numerous academics have puzzled how generally applied the term mental toughness is and the fact that it is one of the least recognized expressions in sport. Until recently, investigations into the phenomena of Mental Toughness were hampered by the widely held belief that Mental Toughness was a "huge cliché" in the sporting world. Today's situation is a little different. Mental toughness is not a new concept, and there have been several applied texts devoted specifically to the development and conceptualization of mental toughness for some time now. The rising academic interest in the Mental Toughness phenomena demonstrates the significance and importance of sport psychologists, coaches, and players on mental toughness. The impact of psychological elements on athletic performance is becoming increasingly essential and visible nowadays, to the point that coaches, athletes, and sports administrators recognize that raw physical talent alone cannot ensure success. Indeed, several researchers have identified mental toughness as a crucial influencing factor in successful performance excellence as well as a performance booster. Although several researchers support this viewpoint, there is still a disturbing lack of conviction in the influence of psychological intervention and its impact on performance in specific circumstances. Researchers employing mental toughness and psychological intervention frameworks are still attempting to capture the trust of a somewhat obstinate audience.

When we face stressful conditions or adversity, the outcome in terms of positive or negative emotional responses and the effects these emotions have on our performance is influenced by our capacity to handle internal and external demands. This refers to the ability to look beyond pure physical talent, skill, and ability into the mental aspect of performance development and optimization. When confronted with challenging performances, too many companies avoid mental elements, and when confronted with circumstances that demand an enhanced level of performance, the spontaneous thought is generally to adjust all levels and phases of their 'physical' training schedule long before the mental element of performance is even regarded. Every athletic contest is a challenge of control, control of the delicate mind-body relationship, yet players continue to train physically at the expense of mental training.

Athletes who can engage in the mental side of training and performance have a significant advantage over those who cannot. The biochemistry of the human body is designed to regulate its basic existence, and this regulation is intimately related to the central control system, the brain and mind. The quality and extent of their psychological preparation and how successfully these athletes apply their skills during high-pressure game conditions can be the deciding factors between a good athlete and a great athlete. It is increasingly critical for athletes who wish to manage the psychological stress of elite sports involvement and sports participation in general. We use the word "mental toughness" as an umbrella phrase for athletes who are thought to have superior mental traits, and they believe that the mental game will differentiate the players. Simply defined, mental toughness distinguishes good from great athletes when physical, technical, and tactical skills are equal. Regardless of physical attributes, the 'tougher' athlete will usually win, and the deciding factor between success and failure is "often more easily, and probably more properly, due to psychological factors."

However, it should be noted that growing and strengthening one's mental side of performance in no way diminishes or trivializes the critical significance of developing and sustaining physical or technical abilities. The idea being made here is that an athlete with physical talent, skill, and ability may become an even better athlete and boost their chances of successful performance and career by beginning to train mentally. An athlete who does not have the same physical ability as other athletes and may be considered significantly weaker in this area may become a better athlete if they learn to engage in mental toughness development, improvement, and maintenance. Athletes frequently refer to the term fitness or a condition of being fit in sports, and the term has many distinct connotations and meanings. In general, an athlete who is deemed fit is in a desired physical condition that allows them to perform at the maximum level possible for their specific role in a certain athletic context. Athletes in modern-day sporting competitions must focus their efforts on becoming mentally fit and achieving a condition of optimal mental fitness. Talent alone does not guarantee success, and there have been cases where highly skilled athletes experienced "burnout" due to a breakdown in mental toughness. In contrast, seemingly less talented athletes thrived at professional levels due to their mental toughness.

Coaches and players alike gradually realize that an additional resource, mental training, is required to stay ahead of the competition. Competitive sports are 85-90 percent a mental game, but regrettably, the physical component of the game is sometimes exaggerated at the expense of the other. The concept of this book is that if athletes and coaches can combine the two parts of mental and technical preparation, they will have a better chance of achieving consistent peak performance every time they compete. They will create a window of opportunity for excellent and elite performance that was previously unexplored, unheard of, and relatively unachievable. They will be venturing into new areas of performance optimization and enhancement. As a result, developing and sustaining mental toughness is critical in today's sporting world, and the difference between success and failure may be defined only by this element.

WHAT IS MENTAL TOUGHNESS

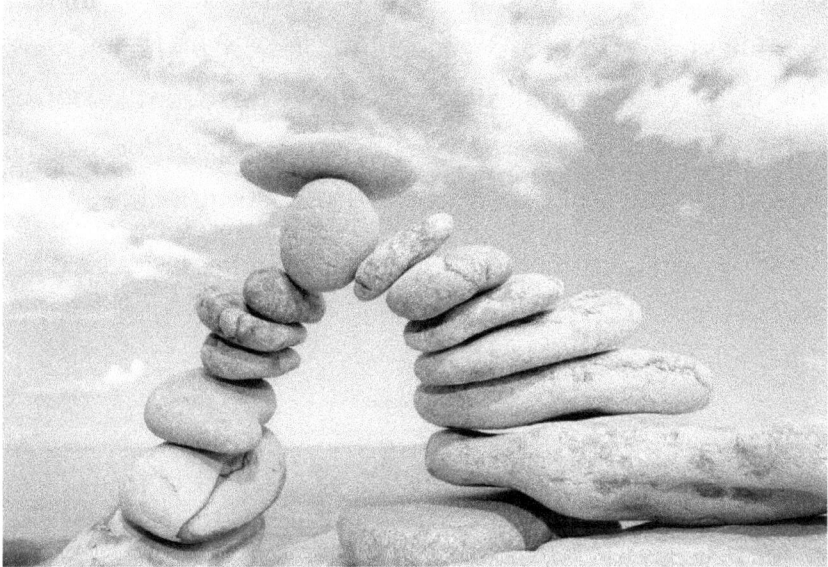

"When the going gets tough, the tough get going."

This is something we've all heard at some point in our lives. Apart from being a sports movie cliché, it also gets to the heart of the rapidly expanding discipline of sport psychology.

Athletes achieve success after thousands of hours of arduous physical training. However, physical ability is not usually what distinguishes professionals from champions at the professional level. Indeed, many professionals are increasingly crediting their success to mental toughness.

When the Patriots defeated the Seahawks in this year's Super Bowl, Tom Brady credited his team's triumph to mental toughness. According to Michael Jordan, mental talents are "the thing that separates the decent players from the great players." "I came in here with the athletic skills," he explained, "but the mental side is the most difficult."

Developing and maintaining mental toughness is critical for understanding and completing tasks in the face of hardship. But what exactly is it?

The concept of mental toughness

The concept of "mental toughness" relates to the ability to overcome disappointments by remaining positive and competitive. It also entails training and preparing oneself psychologically for whatever obstacle may come our way. Staying mentally strong will offer us the grit we need to deal with our mistakes or poor performance and equip us with the tenacity to keep going in the face of them. When things don't go as planned (or the way we want them to), we must maintain our focus and resolve. We must continue to persevere in the face of adversity, which is the exact definition of mental fortitude.

Making routines, using visualization techniques, and practicing self-talk are all ways to improve mental toughness.

Routines

Routines assist us in trusting the process rather than focusing on the outcome. By developing a pre-, during-, and post-performance routine, you avoid one of the most harmful activities a performer may engage in: thinking! Thinking is a crucial component of strategizing before a play, and in some cases, thinking through a game situation during a play is necessary. However, thinking inhibits us from being present in the moment and trusting our natural talent and well-honed skills. A detailed routine can assist most performers and athletes in doing what most coaches would yell at us from the sidelines, "Relax! Slow down the game and stay in the moment!" A routine can help you do this by allowing you to focus on a series of phrases or activities that will center you and prevent you from overthinking.

Visualization

According to elite performers, visualization is critical in maintaining and enhancing mental toughness before and during competitions. Mark Plaatjes, a gold medalist marathon runner, swears by visualization and mental imagery. His triumph in the 1993 World Championships Marathon demonstrates that it has incredible results. Plaatjes was able to win with just three minutes to spare by studying images of the course and utilizing visualization techniques to visualize himself running the track many times before the event. The power of visualization, particularly in athletic training, is mind-boggling, and it is clear how beneficial it can be when people apply it effectively. Using visualization appropriately is obviously subjective, as different ways benefit different people. What worked for Mark Plaatjes may not work the same way for someone else. Regardless of individual variances, it is critical to picture positive outcomes while keeping realistic and expecting the unexpected (good or bad). Visualizations should be detailed and define precisely what you intend to achieve, with space for error and changes in plans in mind. Finally, even though the chances are stacked against you, stay confident and calm and hope for the best.

Maintaining confidence may appear simple, especially before a race or competition, but it is often more complicated than it appears when the pressure and stakes are high. In reality, it's very simple to become frustrated as an athlete, especially if your performance hasn't met your expectations.

Techniques for Self-Talk

Self-talk tactics have been demonstrated to boost confidence and mental toughness in various settings, from the workplace to the court, track, or field.

Individuals can improve their performance by reframing criticisms and using motivational self-talk. Personal affirmations ("I am mentally tough"), a list of accomplishment reminders ("I won first place last year"), and personal pep talks ("I can do this") might help to build mental toughness during lapses in self-confidence and inspire endurance and drive. It is crucial to highlight that realistic self-talk is the most effective. For instance, "I can beat this opponent because I have this pitch in my arsenal." This is more powerful than saying, "I will beat this guy."

Everyone strives to be as physically strong as a professional athlete, but mental toughness allows those few exceptional athletes to excel. Controlling the mental component of performance can increase confidence and an overall clearer and calmer state of mind, ideally resulting in the favorable results you seek. Mental toughness growth, like physical training, will not be simple at first, but with practice, success is guaranteed.

Characteristics of mental toughness

For many years, mental toughness has been discussed in sports literature. Indeed, because of the alignment and common framework it bears, mental toughness has been linked to both the corporate and sporting worlds. This blog discusses ten major traits of mental toughness in athletes.

Ability to recover from defeat - Sports performers will face defeat. Champion athletes such as Michael Phelps, Novak Djokovic, Lionel Messi, and Lewis Hamilton have all been defeated. Elite performers, on the other hand, have an inbuilt aptitude to recover. The ability to bounce back is critical for regaining enthusiasm and self-confidence. Performers access their deep inner sanctums and respond to defeat by fueling their fire for future triumph. In other words, defeat is painful enough for them to recover.

Resilience - A resilient performer will approach each assignment with enthusiasm in order to attain the end goal. The term "resilience" refers to recovering from adversity and improving one's ability to cope with difficulties. Resilience is a trait that performers can employ to boost their self-confidence through the application of mental skills. Tennis players who come back from a two-set deficit during championships are a good example of resilience.

Consistency - Performers must be consistent and stable in their performance and training. The driving principle is linked to habit formation, and the more you perform something (for example, a free throw in basketball), the better you should become. Consistency in your own sport also entails mental and physical preparation.

Composed - Sport is full of emotions that can affect and impact outcomes. The goal of composure is to allow performers to complete tasks with maximum application and little energy consumption. For example, before a gymnastic routine can be successfully done, the mind and body must be in balance. Unsuccessful performers may be fearful of the outcome that leads to failure. Nervousness and tension will only cause the body to tighten and the mind to become confused.

Motivation - It goes without saying that champion athletes require both innate and external motivation. Inner self-belief is essential since it defines desire and commitment. Extrinsic motivation can be used to influence choices based on this inner self-belief. The ability to define process-related goals and achieve them efficiently is essential for motivation.

Confidence - Given the nature of sports and their unpredictability, confidence is essential. Several models guide the purpose of confidence. In summary, confidence refers to being conscious that you can attain a specific goal or do a specific skill. When there is self-doubt, confidence levels are low. Levels of confidence rise when a performer develops self-efficacy.

Desire - Desire and the willingness to succeed are intimately related to confidence. An inner feeling also produces a desire that achievement is possible. Positive body language is visible when teams have set goals and believe they can reach them. Poor body language, on the other hand, has the opposite effect when teams are disconnected.

Organized - In order to reach their goals, top performers are always organized. The organization is dependent on several factors, some of which are subtle but equally vital. Being organized entails planning ahead of time and arriving on time. Following and comprehending key instructions is also essential. A well-organized performer, for example, is more likely to be prepared and focused on the task at hand.

Attention to detail - This is a crucial characteristic of great achievers. It is evident that exceptional athletes (performers or coaches) can identify something tactically far faster than others. Because professional athletics has such tiny margins, attention to detail becomes critical. Indeed, there is evidence of the usage of GPS systems in several team sports to determine how much ground performers have traveled.

Determined - Performers who want to succeed must be determined. Inner self-belief creates determination. Performers achieve achievement and find ways to advance to the next level via determination. Cristiano Ronaldo, New Zealand All Blacks, and the Indian Test Team are recent instances of motivated performers who have successfully advanced to the next level.

Reflective practice is built into mental toughness. To put it another way, to be mentally tough, one should engage in reflective practice, which allows one to appraise one's strengths and work on areas for improvement. Goal setting is a frequent technique for aligning this potential. Mental toughness, reflective practice, and mental skills all work together to support and promote performance.

Personality traits that make you mentally though

Mental toughness indicates that you are capable of dealing with life's challenges. It denotes your ability to function under duress. In recent years, this topic has been the subject of several research studies.

For example, a 2019 study investigated the association between various personality factors that influence our mental toughness. The authors analyzed elite athletes and discovered five personality qualities that predicted athletic achievement.

In this post, I'll discuss the characteristics that make players mentally tough. While their conclusions are not particularly solid or applicable to everyday life, I found their list of five personality traits to be really useful. We can utilize these characteristics as a guideline to improve our mental toughness.

Ego-Strength

I appreciate that the study's authors brought up the connection between ego and mental toughness. The study defines ego as "a measure of one's ability to deal with failures, criticism, and rejection." Ego, in my opinion, is a useful instrument that we should not suppress.

If you have a high ego-strength score, you will be less impacted by failure and setbacks. Failure, criticism, and rejection all have an impact on those who score low. And you'll have a difficult time recovering.

The ego has received a lot of unfavorable attention in recent years. Famous people have made public shows of hubris and ego. Ryan Holiday even penned a book titled "Ego is the Enemy." That book appeals to me because it demonstrates the dangers of having a large ego. But we can't deny that ego can be valuable. Indeed, the study mentioned above found a link between mental toughness and ego-strength.

Here's the takeaway: don't be frightened to embrace your ego. Try to be more inspired by Michael Jordan than Lance Armstrong when they were at their peak. The former exploited his ego to win, while the latter used it to ruin and manipulate others.

Whatever occurs in life, you must have faith in yourself. This isn't woo-woo or self-help nonsense. A competent competitor's basic characteristic is self-belief.

In life, we all fail. We are all losers. We are all subjected to rejection and criticism. But none of this should derail our will to keep moving forward.

Level-Headedness

Mentally tough sportsmen maintain their composure under stressful conditions. This is an important aspect of mental toughness. When confronted with a situation that causes your heart rate to rise, you want to avoid an emotional reaction.

This is a trait in which I naturally rank low. During stressful situations, I frequently became emotional. But after a while, I became bored of it and resolved to control my feelings. Take it from me: you can be more composed if you want to. All you have to do is practice. I write a lot about keeping my cool, and I'm still not where I want to be, but I'm getting there.

Whatever others say to you, what happens to you, or what kind of scenario you're in, you should always maintain your cool. Emotional outbursts will only injure you and others.

Stress-Tolerance

This quality refers to your ability to deal with high-risk situations. How do you handle the possibility of bad consequences? For example, if you have a high-stress tolerance, you are fine with taking the game-winning shot.

If you take the shot consciously, you will almost certainly face an avalanche of negativity if you miss it. I also see folks in finance that have a high-stress tolerance. Assume you are in charge of millions of dollars of other people's money. You can't be overly concerned about the negative repercussions since it will paralyze you.

This is the idea behind stress tolerance. In this scenario, I believe there is a genetic propensity. Some folks have no qualms about making such calls. Others do not want to be held accountable.

That is neither good nor harmful. Not everyone requires or desires to be the person who takes the decisive shot. However, we don't want to be at the bottom of the stress tolerance scale when it comes to mental toughness.

This is a crucial component of living a good life, in my opinion. To avoid anxiety and stress, I employ ideas from ancient philosophy. Stoicism is excellent for this, as is mindfulness. Whatever occurs, don't let the dread of negative repercussions paralyze you.

Energy/Persistence

According to the study, this is "a measure of one's ability to sustain a high level of activity over extended periods." This is the most difficult challenge in my life and at work, in my opinion.

Our energy levels fluctuate far too frequently. As a consequence, even if we wanted to, we cannot be persistent. However, most things in life need long-term effort before we get any kind of benefit.

Consider learning a skill, obtaining a degree, establishing a profession, writing a book, producing a film, and so on. All of that needs effort and perseverance. Consistency, in my opinion, is the most vital factor.

It doesn't matter how fast you can go or how good you are at anything. It is about making consistent growth. You'd like to "chisel away" at something. Consider it as though you were tearing down a wall. Destroy it gradually so as not to tire yourself out. Even with a sledgehammer, going at it with force will simply tire you out.

The trick is to control our energy so that we can remain active and persistent in our efforts to overcome our obstacles.

Thoroughness

For many people, this is one of the major obstacles. "My biggest flaw is that I'm a perfectionist," someone once said during a job interview. That's right, brilliance! In my professional experience, the majority of people are the polar opposite.

We can all be more meticulous and meticulous. I used to speed through things and frequently ignore details. To some extent, I still prefer to move quickly in life. I built and released an online course in five weeks last month. Normally, this process takes twice as long.

However, mental toughness is more than just doing your work; it is also about doing it properly. And in order to achieve in life, you must be thorough. You don't earn points for shoddy work.

The issue arises when we go too far. But, once again, is there such a thing as performing an overly good job? No, I don't think so. When you look at successful people in sports and business, you will see that they have a keen eye for detail.

Steve Jobs is one of the most well-known instances. He was well-known for improving the interiors of their products — parts that we, as users, would never see. The same could be said for Apple's production facilities. Everything had to be immaculate. It's a personality attribute. It's a way of seeing the world. People like Jobs will never settle for less than the best. That is something I admire and find a lot of inspiration in.

<u>Accept Challenges</u>

People frequently ask me, "But how can I improve these characteristics?" Here's my honest response: there are no universal solutions. There is no manual for developing mental toughness. It isn't math. Nobody can tell you, "Do XYZ, and you'll be mentally tough from now on!" Based on what I have observed, simply being aware of these characteristics is enough to get things started. So, if you're looking for specific directions, I wouldn't waste my time on it.

In the end, none of these characteristics will ensure success. That is not the point of this. I utilized the attributes listed above to define various facets of mental toughness, and everyone has their life purpose and path. Everyone does not have to be like Michael Jordan.

Mental toughness is also unrelated to results. It's all about pushing yourself and becoming a better — and more complete — person. I hope these characteristics provided you with adequate topics to concentrate on. I recommend focusing on one or two characteristics in your daily life.

Mental toughness vs. mental strength

These two expressions are frequently used interchangeably, particularly in the media and among people development professionals.

However, we tend to be cautious about how we label mental toughness for a handful of crucial reasons.

To begin, the inverse of Mental Toughness is Mental Sensitivity. Mental Weakness is the polar opposite of Mental Strength. These are not synonymous.

It is generally true that the mentally tough have an advantage – they tend to achieve more, have better well-being, are more positive, and even earn more – whereas the mentally sensitive find the road through life and work more difficult – they can feel every bump in the road and the consequences that come with it.

However, we should not think that there are no exceptions. In my consulting experience, I have met mentally sensitive people who have succeeded and achieved great results and other mentally tough people who have failed in their goals and are always dissatisfied.

The key to success is self-awareness. Whether you are mentally tough or mentally sensitive, being self-aware of who you are and why you think the way you do is the key to being able to do something about your collection of traits.

The second reason is just as significant. Across the mental toughness scale, there are potential strengths and weaknesses. Although the mentally sensitive may be vulnerable to disadvantages and have deficiencies in terms of their goals, studies show that they also have attributes that we would call strengths.

They are frequently more aware of possible overload and burnout, which is useful in team settings. They can be more collaborative – they tend to have lower degrees of goal orientation, which means they can be successful followers – it is less likely that their aims will be misaligned with yours if you are the leader. And they are frequently creative - because they observe and think about the world from a distinct perspective, which they bring to their work. Consider artists and musicians!

Similarly, the mentally tough has potential flaws. A high level of control might lead to the mindset of "I can do it, why can't you?" which isn't always useful. With the Commitment factor, it is possible to overcommit and burn out without recognizing exhaustion signals.

When it comes to challenging, they can overdo it, finally taking too many risks and sometimes being lured by the next "new" thing before they sort out what they are working on. And because of the Confidence factor, they may be overconfident in their Abilities. When they are Interpersonally Confident, they might drown out the contributions of others, emerging as "verbal bullies" in severe cases.

As difficult as it is for the mentally sensitive. Much of our work is with senior executives who have risen to positions of prominence – frequently through mental toughness – and then discover that they are not as effective as they would like to be, particularly in engaging with others.

As a result, self-awareness, contemplation, and focused development are essential for everyone.

When we look at people, the world isn't black and white; there are many colors and variances. The mental toughness idea contributes significantly to the understanding and developing personalities, whether we are talking about ourselves or others.

THE PSYCHOLOGY OF MENTAL TOUGHNESS

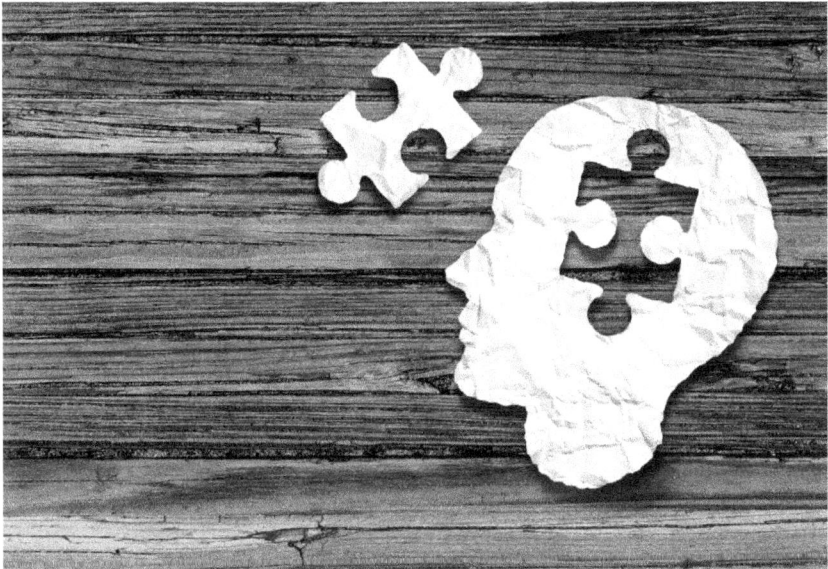

When people feel overwhelmed, out of control, or unable to take effective action, they frequently seek therapy. They believe they have come to work things out and may be unaware that counseling might help them become stronger. Making decisions and carrying them out requires more than just willpower.

How does it work?

Life throws us unexpected curveballs, such as a worldwide recession that knocks decent enterprises out of business. This becomes your concern when you learn that your 20-year employer is closing down next week. Your whole world - the one you've always believed in - has been turned upside down. You're at a loss for what to do. You catch your breath and are confronted with frightening options. Do you give up your job? Take whatever job you can get? Return to school for additional training? Should you downsize to a smaller house?

You (like many others) may find it tough to pick up the phone to get things started and dismiss yourself as "weak" or "lazy." You lack the "get up and go" to complete the task. Perhaps you force yourself to behave. Why was it so difficult even back then? Are you really that sluggish? And how do you get around that?

A matter for the tough

Our cultural ideal is to be resilient in the face of misfortune. It is an ideal since it is not something that everyone can achieve. It's also all too easy to dismiss fortitude under duress as a skill that you either have or don't. However, there are few absolutes in our daily world. Most people handle some situations well while becoming overwhelmed by others. Can you improve your capacity to keep your cool under duress? Absolutely! Let's look at how you can train your mind to be tough in the face of adversity.

Consider an Olympic decathlete who competes in ten events that test strength, ability, and endurance over the course of two days. A decathlete's training cannot ignore any of these characteristics and requires time to succeed. Otherwise, they will succeed at shot put but struggle at javelin throw and 1500 meter run. Similarly, if you want to grow mental muscle, you should focus on your strengths while strengthening your deficiencies.

A person with mental toughness confronts obstacles head-on and effectively solves them. Someone who is mentally tough, in my opinion, possesses a combination of willpower, skill, and resilience. How can treatment assist you in developing these qualities? Let's have a look at the many aspects of mental toughness and how they are addressed in psychotherapy.

An experienced therapist will examine your individual requirements and use tried-and-true methods to help you. Growth does not normally happen in a straight line but rather through a process of trial and error through time. Therapy can assist you in pacing and tracking this process. The therapist's responsibility is to explain a treatment plan that includes goals, procedures, timetables, and fees.

Developing mental toughness through therapy

Willpower is defined as a combination of intention, effort, and courage.

The "will" in willpower refers to intention. It is the determination to stay on task or return to it until the work is completed. To help you become more aware of what may be required, your therapist can help you clarify your values so that you can make decisions that are consistent with them.

You can also investigate the repercussions of changing behavior - what you might fear losing as well as what you might gain – so that when you're ready, you can change on your own terms.

The effort is power, and it is strengthened by assisting you in precisely gauging the quantity required. If you are confronted with a significant problem, you may be afraid, helpless, or sad about taking it on. In this case, your therapist will address your susceptibility to anxiety or sadness so that you do not stall. If you give up quickly, you may bring to the surface the thoughts or prior experiences that make you feel terrified, helpless, and hopeless, and then explore alternative points of view. You'll be encouraged by the therapist's encouragement and support the entire time.

Courage is the ability to tolerate the intensity of fear and other emotions while yet doing what needs to be done. Awareness is a necessary component of courage. Newer cognitive behavior treatments teach people how to be mindful to improve their ability to witness their experiences and act in their best interests despite discomforts and distractions.

How anxiety and depression are related

When under stress, some people become nervous, while others become depressed, or these feed off each other, causing coping skills to halt.

The nervous reaction

When confronted with a challenging challenge, you get so worried that you lose focus on the subject at hand. Your terror takes center stage and overwhelms you. As a result, you distance yourself from the dread and the situation.

The depressive reaction

You tell yourself that it is hopeless; therefore, you feel helpless. This de-energizes you exactly when you need to be positive.

How do anxiety and depression interact?

Fearful thoughts tell you that the situation is hopeless, so you avoid difficulties, causing issues to worsen. Responding to stress with an escape – whether through drinking, watching TV, or other behaviors – reinforces the perception that you lack willpower. You are now embarrassed and guilty, and you have lost faith in yourself, so you avoid the pain, and the cycle continues.

Seeking counseling is one of the options for reversing this negative cycle. It is going beyond oneself in order to strengthen your coping skills and feel better. Even in this case, acknowledging you need help may have an impact on your self-esteem.

You don't have to stay stuck in such negativity. The first step is to confess to yourself that you are overwhelmed. Then gather your power and seek assistance from someone who is competent, trustworthy, and capable of assisting you in marshaling your abilities to tackle obstacles more effectively.

Behavioral therapists teach clients how to develop their ability to relax and access that relaxation in otherwise uncomfortable situations, allowing them to be "cool under fire." Psychodynamic and other therapists encourage you to share your experiences without fear of repercussions. They work with you to explore the challenging emotions and thoughts that arise, sometimes tracing their origins to earlier events, which can help you let go of their grip. Methods that address the intensity of emotional discomforts, such as Eye Movement Desensitization Reprocessing (EMDR), have you examine traumatic experiences in the safety of the consulting room and help free you from panic responses that such memories frequently accompany.

In the depths of the 1930s Great Depression, Franklin Delano Roosevelt stood at the inaugural podium on withered knees braced with steel braces and declared, "The only thing we have to fear is fear itself." How do you cultivate this kind of bravery? You gradually overcome your fear by addressing it and doing what you need to do nonetheless.

For example, if you're frightened of driving over bridges, you could avoid any route that includes one. Your therapist may teach you how to relax by doing slow, deep belly breathing or showing you how to tension and relax your muscles. He may also introduce you to exposure treatment, which involves practicing calm breathing while observing the bridge from a distance. You can then drive near an actual bridge while practicing relaxation until you've calmed down enough to drive over it. You can begin the exposure process by picturing the circumstance from afar, then closer, which prepares you for the actual situation.

Skill

Skill is a blend of awareness, thinking, and perspective. Attention and focus are examples of awareness. These are produced by investigating the problems that are causing them and becoming aware of what may be contributing to them. Whereas life stress causes intense emotions, you may be taught in meditation, which teaches you how to concentrate or conduct everyday activities thoughtfully rather than fumbling your way through them. Journal writing, focusing on your feelings until you have a deeper intuition about what they're expressing, and dreamwork, where your associations may bring insight into your attitude and life situation, are all methods that can help you become more conscious.

Brain dysfunctions considered disabling, such as severe depression, bipolar disease, or attention deficit hyperactivity disorder, can impede attention and focus (ADHD). Medication can be extremely beneficial in certain cases. Substance misuse, which needs to be addressed, may also decrease awareness.

Escape from avoidance

Some people become locked in a subtle form of avoidance in which they appear to be doing something but are only doing it half-heartedly and in a stupor. For example, rather than responding to his wife's request to converse, a husband goes to his computer and spends hours surfing the Internet. Or, a young woman loses herself in trashy literature but feels unable to get her life in order. This haven can take many different forms. It is neither fully active nor wholly unconscious, and it gives the impression that you are doing something, yet it produces nothing except emptiness.

If you find yourself in this state of sluggishness, you should first recognize that you are there. Then get up and go on to something else. Look at what you were avoiding and handle it immediately if possible, or examine what you're avoiding if you're still stuck. However, get out of that swamp because it is one of the ways to become trapped in sadness.

Thinking

Cognitive therapists employ automatic thought logs to assist you in training your awareness and thinking. This is how they work: You are thrown off guard by a scenario. You write down what happened as soon as possible and analyze the thoughts sparked by the circumstance to see if those thoughts are a distorted account of what you observed. Then you write down the sentiments evoked by those thoughts and assess their strength. Then you converse with those thoughts to discover a more adaptive reaction. You conclude by quantifying the level of emotions that are now associated with that experience.

Often, you'll notice that your emotional response has cooled significantly, allowing you to respond in a more adaptable manner in the future. Similar benefits can be obtained by discussing such experiences, thoughts, emotions, and potential answers with your therapist. She may also engage you in role-play to help you gain confidence and learn new abilities. All of these techniques help you think more clearly under pressure. Inherited learning and attention impairments, such as dyslexia, may exist in some people. Your therapist may send you for evaluation and include such concerns in your treatment plan.

Perspective

Perspective is the ability to step back from a situation and consider it in context. A solution-focused therapist may be able to help you picture the life you desire and begin doing the things that will lead to it. Dreamwork, art therapy, and sand tray therapy are all imaginative approaches that allow you to work with pictures that come to you spontaneously. These and similar strategies assist you in seeing that your unconscious mind already has the broader viewpoint you seek.

The most common way for gaining perspective is talk therapy. Your therapist may assist you in exploring your circumstance and the numerous factors that contribute to them. Interpreting your actions through the prism of unresolved childhood issues might sometimes assist you in understanding responses that no longer make sense. You may also benefit from prescribed reading and discussion of research findings relevant to your situation.

Resilience

Staying power necessitates resilience, which may be defined as a combination of patience, flexibility, self-care, and support.

Patience

Patience can help you avoid compounding difficulties and more effectively pace your responses. It is taught by encouraging students to set realistic goals. If you undertake meditation practice, you will improve your capacity to stay focused in the face of distractions or discomfort, and you will be able to maintain your focus for a longer time. People who are so impatient that they frequently perform rash, impulsive behaviors may need to learn emotion management and discomfort tolerance skills, or they may need to stop fueling addictions.

Anger might sometimes cause impulsive behavior. Those who are prone to rage can benefit from anger management programs and training to help them assert themselves more effectively, taking into account the needs of others as well as their own.

Flexibility

The readiness to adapt your action plan when circumstances change is referred to as flexibility. It all starts with gaining a clear vision of your problem and considering alternate routes of action. Several therapy methods, such as dialog, role play, problem-solving, and communication skills training, promote flexibility.

Self-care

When people are stressed, self-care is crucial since the mind has a body! Physical health gives you the stamina to deal with stress. Many people find that starting regular exercise, eating healthier meals, and learning proven strategies to deal with insomnia helps to lighten their depression (or seeking medical help if insomnia continues). People may also stay in tough situations or relationships until they can fix them or move on. A skilled therapist will assist you in accomplishing this.

Compassion for oneself is one of the most crucial aspects of self-care because few individuals prefer to be trapped. They usually do their best with the knowledge and resources they have. Your therapist will assist you in auditing your self-care practices and identifying medical conditions whose symptoms may mimic mental illness. Licensed therapists are trained to detect this risk and refer you for a medical evaluation. Self-care must include the resolution of addictions that inhibit full healing, just as it must include the development of other strengths.

We all require assistance since we are stronger as a group than as individuals. Building a support network may entail assisting you in planning and gaining access to the most useful people of your family and community, including your therapist and other treatment team members.

Support

Support groups or group therapy can help certain people. In addition, if you are under a lot of stress or if your discovery process becomes so active that you need more time to digest your changes, your therapist may suggest more frequent sessions.

You've now gone over the characteristics that comprise mental toughness. You've also seen how your therapist can assist you in doing the difficult work that builds individual strengths. Building a more optimistic attitude and hope that you can conquer even the most severe obstacles is one of the benefits of a successful course of therapy. Achieving mental toughness is a gift that will last for the rest of your life.

WHY MENTAL TOUGHNESS IS SO IMPORTANT

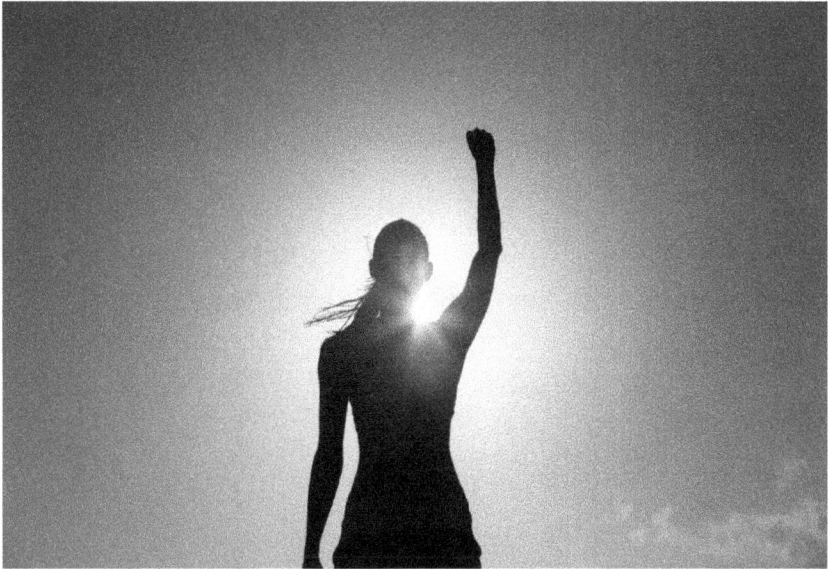

Mental toughness describes the mindset that everyone adopts in everything they do, and it is necessary and helpful for everyone on two levels.

For starters, it explains why people and organizations act the way they do. Personality can be defined as someone's distinctive style of thinking, feeling, and acting, and it can explain individual differences as well as how people behave in given situations.

Mental toughness is a personality trait that characterizes a person's mindset. It investigates what is going on in the mind of the individual to explain why they behave the way they do.

Mindset and behavior

As a result, there is an evident connection between mindset and behavior. Mindset can be described as both a precursor to behavior and an explanation for such behavior.

Second, research and case studies from around the world reveal that Mental Toughness is a significant component in the majority of key outcomes for individuals and organizations:

Performance

Individual differences in performance can account for up to 25% of the range in performance.

Mentally tough people produce more, work more meaningfully, demonstrate more remarkable dedication to purpose, and are more competitive. This leads to higher output, on-time and on-budget deliveries, and improved attendance.

Happiness — feeling more content.

Mentally tough people have better stress management, better attendance, are less likely to develop mental health concerns, sleep better, and are less likely to be bullied. They are capable of dealing with stress.

Positive Behaviour – more involved

Mentally tough people are more cheerful, have more "can-do" attitudes, respond positively to change and hardship, have better attendance, are more likely to contribute to a positive culture, embrace responsibility, and volunteer for new chances and activities.

Openness to Learning – more aspirational

Mentally tough people are more ambitious and willing to take on more danger.

Being mentally tough has several advantages for both individuals and organizations. According to global research, persons with higher levels of mental toughness, as measured by the MTQ48, receive the following benefits:

Better performance — it accounts for up to 25% of the variation in job performance.

Increased positivism — adopting a more "can do" attitude, leading to increased rapport and connectivity with coworkers.

Increased well-being — more happiness and better stress management.

Change management is a more relaxed and stress-free approach to organizational change.

Increased desire and confidence in reaching goals and a higher readiness to endure to do so.

For these reasons, being mentally robust is critical for an individual or an organization, especially during times of extreme upheaval. Leaders, aspiring leaders, and individuals working in stressful, unforgiving occupations and uncertainty or dynamic change situations require mental toughness.

Organizations in the education, health, government, corporate, and public sectors must be resilient and mentally prepared for change.

Benefits of training mental toughness

When we look at successful people, we often wonder how they did it and their secret to success. We may believe it is due to their talents, abilities, and knowledge, but mental power is even more important. We all have mental strength, albeit to varying degrees. Because you know how to deal with and overcome challenging situations, mental strength provides you the ability to work hard and always go forward. You will be able to achieve your goals and be successful if you teach yourself to be more mentally tough.

1. Mental fortitude can assist you in filtering out unhelpful comments and recommendations.

Caring about what other people think and their ideas and suggestions can significantly impact our choices, forcing us to lose our own identity to satisfy others. If you are mentally strong, you will be able to focus entirely on your goal and adhere to your principles while ignoring unpleasant and unhelpful comments.

2. Mental toughness can help you recover from failure.

Failure is unavoidable in our life, but how we deal with them reveals how mentally strong we are. Whereas some people might just quit up after a failure, those who are psychologically strong see it as an important lesson on the way to success and rapidly recover.

3. Emotional regulation can be aided by mental fortitude.

We experience many emotions on our route to success, and if we don't learn how to regulate them, they will affect our actions and lead us astray. By developing mental strength, you may gain control over your emotions and avoid allowing them to influence your actions.

4. Mental toughness can give you the courage to face your anxieties.

We don't like being put in unfamiliar situations and out of our comfort zone, but being mentally strong allows you to be confident enough to tolerate the discomfort and face your concerns. Only by consistently pushing yourself and confronting your worries will you be able to grow toward achievement.

5. Mental fortitude can help you maintain a strong sense of self-worth.

Whatever objective you are attempting to attain, at some point along the way, you will most certainly begin to doubt yourself and if you are good enough or capable enough to achieve it. Mentally strong people understand how much they are worth, and when confronted with such situations, they are self-assured enough to shut out the voice of doubt and continue with great self-esteem.

6. Mental fortitude can help you stay motivated.

Everything goes more smoothly when you are motivated, but what happens when you reach a snag and your motivation drops? How do you react when you lose sight of why you're doing something and want to abandon it all? That is where mental fortitude comes in handy. It encourages you to keep going even when you don't think you have the strength to do so. It helps you rediscover your inner strength and reminds you of your ultimate aim.

7. Mental strength can assist you in learning from your mistakes.

When we commit a mistake, many of us try to find an excuse to justify our behavior to avoid feeling guilty, which is wrong. When we justify our mistakes in order to minimize our guilt, we set ourselves up to repeat them. Mental fortitude allows you to admit that you are to blame for your faults. Admitting to yourself that you were mistaken can help you avoid repeating the same error in the future, which is a useful lesson that will help you progress.

Ten signs you are mentally strong

As a psychotherapist and author of books about mental strength, I encounter many misconceptions about being mentally strong.

Many of the acts that are commonly associated with weakness are, in fact, signs of strength. Our culture frequently places a premium on "toughness" over "real strength."

Acting tough is all about outward looks. It entails constructing a persona that persuades others that you are immune to pain.

Working on your character is essential for true mental strength. Mentally strong people may seem to be vulnerable, and their openness and honesty are frequently misinterpreted as fragility.

Here are ten characteristics of mental strength that are frequently misunderstood as flaws:

<u>To be kind</u>

Many individuals appear to believe that being kind equates to being a pushover or a people pleaser. However, caring for a neighbor, giving a colleague the benefit of the doubt, and volunteering your time to help someone with a project can all be signs of strength.

Kindness frequently necessitates bravery and self-assurance. What if the recipient declines your assistance? What if your gesture of friendship isn't returned? Strong people are not afraid to take those social risks.

Changing your mind

Changing your views does not necessarily imply that you are wishy-washy or readily swayed. Instead, it could signal that you're open to learning more and hearing new views.

Whether your political views have evolved over time or your beliefs have transformed as you've gotten older, altering your mind could be evidence that you're maturing and learning.

Recognizing and accepting your flaws

There is a distinction to be made between telling the truth and putting yourself down. Recognizing that you're awful at facing people or that you struggle with an organization may demonstrate that you're brave enough to admit your flaws.

Recognizing your flaws might also help you take effective action. You might delegate tasks that you struggle with, or you could devise a strategy to help you achieve despite your flaws.

Being patient

With so much focus these days on "hustle," patience is frequently misconstrued with laziness or a lack of desire.

However, large ambitions, such as getting out of debt or getting in shape, necessitate patience. True change does not come overnight, and it requires strength to maintain the patience required to get there.

Seeking assistance

Saying "I can't do this on my own" takes a lot of guts. Whether you approach your supervisor for more aid or a mental health expert, asking for help involves humility and character strength.

Mentally strong people do not go alone. They encircle themselves with people who can help them along the journey.

Failing

If you are successful in whatever you do, it suggests you are living well inside your comfort zone. Making mistakes and failing implies you're pushing yourself, which is an obvious indicator of strength.

Don't allow someone to persuade you that your failures prove you aren't strong enough to succeed. Instead, see failure as proof that you're pushing yourself as far as you can.

Expressing your feelings

Some people are eager to express their anger, but lying beneath those angry sensations are more unpleasant emotions such as sadness, shame, and disappointment. However, it is frequently easier to declare "You're an idiot" than "My sentiments are wounded."

Labeling your emotions and figuring out how to express them in a healthy way takes courage. It's far easier to suppress your pain or try to persuade others that you're perfect.

Giving up

Giving up a goal because the effort required to achieve it isn't a high priority or walking away from a heated argument because you know nothing productive will happen doesn't imply you're giving up.

In reality, it takes courage to walk away from something that isn't working, especially when you've invested all your time and energies into it (or a person). However, walking away may demonstrate that you are willing to act in accordance with your ideals, even if it may result in ridicule.

Improving yourself

Some individuals roll their eyes when they see someone reading a self-help book (usually the same folks who mock overweight people for going to the gym). However, bettering yourself — physically, spiritually, or emotionally — is a difficult task.

Attempting to become a better person demonstrates your desire to effect positive change in your life. Whether you join a support group, go to counseling, visit spiritual retreats, or listen to self-help podcasts, a desire for self-growth is a sign of strength.

Keeping your cool

"Isn't it amazing how she just stood there? I would have told him what was on my mind!" Such remarks indicate that persons who remain calm lack the confidence to advocate for themselves.

The ability to control one's emotions is a sign of mental power. That isn't to imply you won't feel angry (anger can be a really healthy and helpful feeling), but it does mean you'll be able to act productively even when you're upset.

HOW TO DEVELOP MENTAL TOUGHNESS

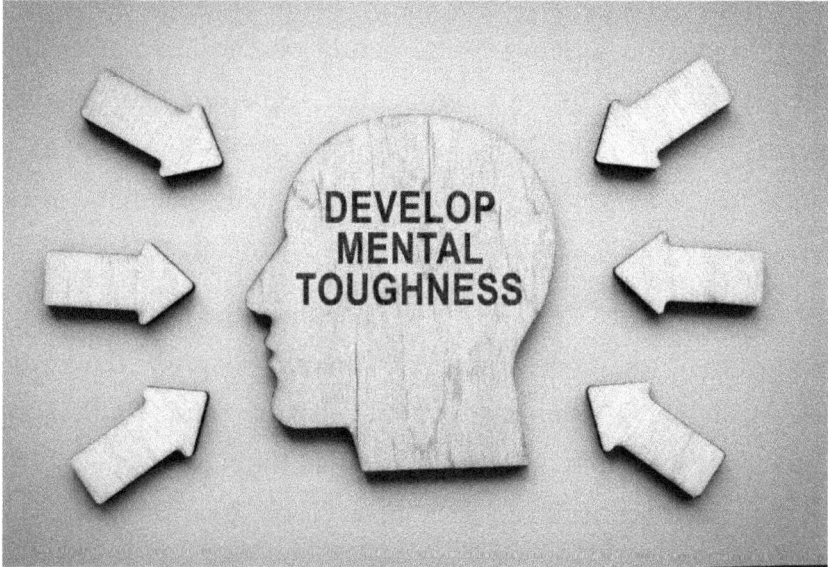

Are you the type of person that aspires to have achievement in life? Do you have the mental toughness to pull it off?

I believe we can all agree that achieving success, regardless of your aspirations, can be challenging, and the daily grind can take a toll on your physical, mental, and emotional stamina over time.

Successful people endure ups and downs on their way to success, including failure, burnout, discouragement, tiredness, self-limiting beliefs, stress, and so much more.

How do some people keep striving for their personal goals year after year while others give up? How can those folks maintain their strength and perseverance when the odds are stacked against them?

According to recent research, mental power is a significant factor in achieving success. The secret to remarkable performance is not talent, but a unique blend of passion and perseverance known as 'grit.'" In other words, when it comes to achieving goals, mental toughness is crucial.

At its most basic, mental toughness is just the ability to stay with something when things get difficult. People with strong levels of mental toughness can overcome these challenges and carve a route to success, whereas others with low levels of mental toughness may give up on their aspirations.

The good news is that you can build the mental toughness you need to be successful regardless of who you are, what you've been told, or what you currently think.

Develop a positive attitude

If you want to enhance your mental toughness and manage stress, the first step is to focus on developing a strong, positive mindset in everyday life.

The average person has 60,000 thoughts every day, according to the Cleveland Clinic. Ninety-five percent of those thoughts reoccur every day, and on average, 80 percent of those recurrent concepts are negative.

That equates to around 45,600 negative thoughts every day!

Carrying these negative thoughts with you is like going on a mountain climb with a rucksack full of boulders. The hike is difficult enough on its own, but adding extra weight is a formula for disaster.

Building mental toughness isn't always about gaining new strength but rather about reserving your strength for the correct tasks. Isn't it easier to just drop the pebbles out of the backpack instead of trying to build up the strength to handle the extra weight?

Let Go of Self-Sacrifice Beliefs

It's difficult to be psychologically tough when you're continuously berating yourself. Any belief that holds you back in any way is considered a self-limiting belief. Following are some examples:

"I'm not clever enough to..."

"I don't have the necessary experience..."

"I tried it before, and it didn't work out, so I must just be awful at..."

When we allow self-limiting thoughts to infiltrate our minds, negative self-talk becomes prevalent, crowding out our ability to think positively.

When you see a self-limiting idea arising in your head, swiftly silence it by telling yourself that it is not true, and then support that with some positive affirmations:

51

"I am intelligent enough; I may just need to do some additional research first."

"I may not have as much experience as someone else, but that will not deter me from trying. I have sufficient experience to get started. I'll sort out the rest on the way."

"Just because I failed the last time doesn't guarantee I'll fail this time. "My past does not determine my future."

Get Rid of the All-or-Nothing Mentality

All-or-nothing thinking is another type of negative thinking that may be hindering you from developing mental toughness.

Extreme thinking is characterized by all-or-nothing thinking. You are either successful or unsuccessful. Your performance was either excellent or dreadful. If you aren't perfect, you are a failure.

But this is not the case!

Isn't dropping 28 pounds better than not losing any weight at all if you're hoping to lose 30? That's what I'd say!

If you allow all-or-nothing thinking to govern your head, you will be ecstatic when you achieve but depressed when you fail. Recognizing the shades of gray in between will enable you to perceive achievement more frequently.

When you notice an all-or-nothing thought, remember to seek the bright side of the circumstance. What have you gained by attempting? <p>What would you miss if you didn't try? What could you have done better if it was your second time?

Ditch the dwelling

Self-limiting ideas and all-or-nothing thinking can lead to harmful dwelling, which is unhealthy for mental health. If you want to boost your mental toughness and keep your mind healthy, you must stop dwelling.

When we linger on our misfortunes, we lose vast quantities of energy that could otherwise be used to attain our objectives. When this happens, we are more prone to give up completely.

That doesn't mean you're not psychologically tough; it simply means you're wasting energy.

Allow yourself to feel disappointed and frustrated the next time something awful happens, but work on limiting the amount of time you linger on the event.

If you're having trouble with this, try the following:

- Call a buddy or a mentor and go over the situation with them. Get a second opinion on your problem.
- Allowing oneself to dwell for no more than one hour will help you to time block your dwelling.
- Then tell yourself to go on, that you're human, that it's okay to make errors or suffer setbacks.

- If everything else fails, find a decent strategy to divert your attention until you can calm down and evaluate the situation with a clear head.

The sooner you can focus on the positives and move past the difficulty, the sooner you will be able to return to your life's success.

Get in tune with your purpose

Having a solid "why" for all of your short and long-term goals is one of the most important aspects of developing mental toughness and maintaining a strong and focused mind.

If you set out to attain a lofty objective without a compelling "why," you will become distracted, frustrated, or disengaged as soon as you face your first setback.

Consider the last time you were working on a goal or resolution that wasn't going well. Perhaps you believed you lacked willpower or discipline.

It's more likely that you simply didn't have a compelling enough reason.

"Your 'why' is the motivation, cause, or belief that drives you."

Pursuing a goal or task for which you have no reason is one of the most draining things you can do to your mental resources. We often set objectives because we like the concept of the goal rather than the reality of the goal. We cannot intrinsically drive ourselves to attain our most difficult goals until we connect to our why.

<u>Discover Intrinsic Motivation</u>

Intrinsic motivation is our intrinsic desire to do something, and it manifests itself when we work toward something that fulfills us above all else — not our parents, bosses, or teachers.

Assume you want to quit smoking because you know it's unhealthy for you, but you really enjoy it. It will be nearly hard to quit smoking if you do not sincerely want to, regardless of your willpower or mental toughness.

However, if you want to quit smoking because you recently had a baby and don't want your child to grow up among smoke, that "why" will provide you with intrinsic drive. Personal motivation is significantly more potent than simple willpower, and it is far easier to sustain over time.

If you're seeking to build mental toughness, attaching a why to everything you want to achieve can lessen the amount of work and energy required to accomplish those goals.

Look for Strength in Unity

The third part of gaining mental toughness is accepting the fact that you are not alone in this.

Bill Gates did not build Microsoft by himself. Steve Jobs did not create the iPhone alone. Oprah did not create her network on her own. Michelle Obama did not launch the "Let's Move" initiative alone.

Some innumerable other people offered support, mentorship, direction, and encouragement to all of these outstanding people.

If you want to acquire unrivaled mental toughness, you must realize that you do not have to go it alone. A team supports even the toughest Navy Seals.

Find a mentor

There are far too many advantages to having a great mentor to name, but to summarize, a mentor is someone who will assist show you the route to success, uncover your best abilities, identify and overcome your blind spots, and work through your limitations.

If you're having trouble dealing with your internal negativity or discovering your purpose, talk it out with a mentor. We can sometimes lose sight of the forest for the trees, and a mentor can help us take a step back and see the larger picture.

Recruit some cheerleaders

It never hurts to have a group of personal cheerleaders to help you achieve your goals if you want to stay strong. Unlike mentors, who would rush in and help you solve your difficulties, a cheerleading squad will help keep your spirits up.

Even if you have a strong why and a good outlook, maintaining a positive mood 100 percent of the time is impossible. It does not make you weak to require assistance from time to time. It makes all the difference in the world to have a group of people cheering you on.

Tell a few close friends what you're doing while you work toward your goals, and when things get rough, tell them about it. When they give you the motivation you need, don't fight it or oppose it with your self-limiting thoughts.

Allow their optimism to recharge your batteries, and then use that energy to keep going.

Create an accountability group

Cheerleaders are lovely, but we need someone to give us the push we need to keep going every now and again. You may have a compelling reason for running a marathon or dropping 30 pounds, but that doesn't imply it will be easy, and forcing yourself to follow through is a sure way to drain your mental energy.

Why not save some of your mental energy by creating a support group?

Find someone or a group of people who share your goals or, at the very least, the need for an accountability partner. Then, make a group commitment to push each other every day.

Learn to get back up after a setback

It is not easy to create a strong mindset and mental toughness! Anyone who has achieved great success understands that hurdles, setbacks, and failure are unavoidable, and you are no exception.

You will have many ups and downs while striving toward your goals, but this does not imply that you lack mental toughness, willpower, or discipline.

Instead of immediately quitting up when you find yourself in a rut, ask yourself the following questions:

- "Am I being overly critical of myself?"
- "Are my negative thoughts affecting my perspective?"
- "What is the silver lining to this setback/obstacle/failure?"
- "What made this objective so essential to me?" "What was my goal?"
- "Does this aim still matter to me?"
- "Who can I turn to for assistance? "Who can coach me or hold me accountable?"

Asking oneself these questions is an excellent approach to assess your current state of mind. It's all too easy to become discouraged when we get caught up in negative thinking or lose sight of our goal.

Bringing it all together

Learning to notice negative tendencies and fix them early on with healthy habits is essential for developing mental toughness. The goal of developing mental toughness is not to eliminate weakness but to learn how to deal with and overcome it.

No one is flawless, but we may cultivate mental toughness worthy of life's most difficult tasks by focusing on the right things.

TEN EXERCISES TO BUILD YOUR MENTAL STRENGTH

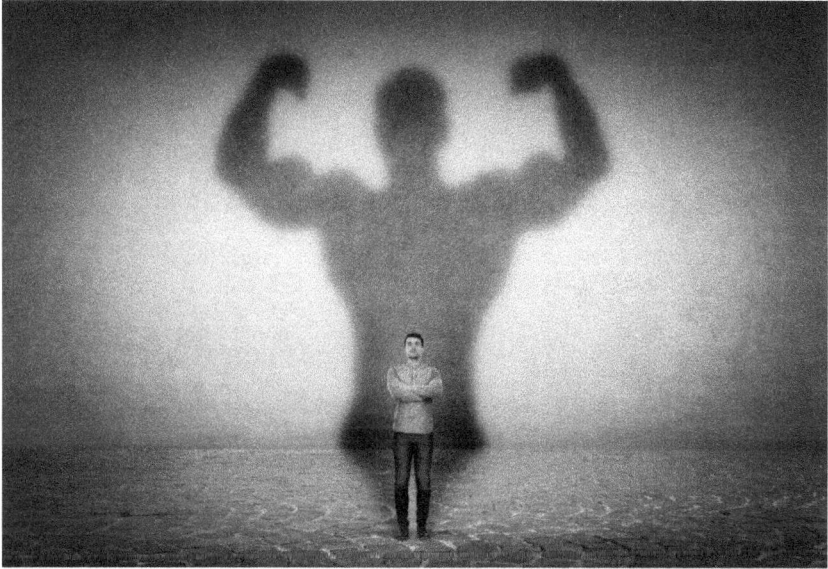

Mental toughness is always necessary. But it isn't a leap to say that everyone could use a little more of it these days. Mental toughness ensures that we don't lose our cool when things don't go our way and avoid physically and emotionally hard situations, just because we can't deal with our emotions. In a nutshell, it's the ability to persevere in terrible conditions, such as the one we're all facing right now, and there are numerous activities you can do to strengthen it, both for yourself and your family.

Suffering helps young troops acquire mental resilience in the military. They'd be in icy lakes of water, staying outside and getting wet - the military has some very strange techniques of breaking down the person. They had to figure out how to deal with difficult situations that drill instructors threw at them. However, there are a variety of mental toughness activities that do not necessitate attending bootcamp.

Throughout my long consulting career, I have identified a variety of exercises to effectively develop mental toughness. While they don't take much time, they will prepare you to be more resilient in times of adversity with practice.

Take cold showers.

Each expert we spoke with the linked mental toughness to the ability to bear the discomfort, whether emotionally or physically. Starting or finishing each day with a cold shower is a simple — albeit difficult — method to become more comfortable with discomfort.

We increase our endocrine function, lymph circulation, which enhances our immune system, and blood circulation when we take cold showers. The cold shower is advised as part of one's daily morning practice in the yogic tradition. It increases blood flow to the capillaries, improves the nervous system, and increases mental fortitude.

I realize it's difficult to step into an ice-cold shower. However, it will provide continual physical and mental resilience training for those willing to take on the challenge and provide a surge of endorphins and energy for the day.

Do you want to take it slowly? I propose holding the handheld shower head over one arm at a time, then one leg at a time, gradually working your way up to the entire body (except the head).

Don't eat as soon as you get hungry

Allowing yourself to feel hungry without reaching for a snack is another basic strategy for increasing tolerance for discomfort (and impulse control).

Tolerating an additional five to ten minutes of hunger improves patience. You can accept that it's okay to wait and be hungry since you know you'll eat. But instead of rushing in to remedy things, you just sit with it. This increases your tolerance for discomfort. If you can achieve that, you'll be able to handle more difficult problems.

Do what you don't like (for 10 minutes)

When you really don't want to do anything, like work out or read a tedious report, tell yourself you just have to do it for 10 minutes. Allow yourself to stop after the 10-minute mark if you want to. (You're probably going to keep going - getting started is usually the most difficult part.)

Starting whatever you don't like to do teaches your brain that you don't have to succumb to your emotions. Just because you don't feel like doing something doesn't mean you can't. You're tougher than you think, and you can act even when you're not motivated.

This also applies to taking on larger challenges. When your mind tries to talk you out of doing something (such as giving a presentation or taking up a new activity), react with, "Mission accomplished."

Your brain undervalues you. But every time you accomplish something you thought you couldn't, you encourage your brain to regard you as more competent than it already does.

Workout in silence

Working out is, without a doubt, an excellent approach to improve both your physical and mental power. However, if you do it while listening to music or watching TV, you are diverting yourself and restricting your ability to feel and build tolerance for discomfort. Switch off your smartphone or tablet and focus on your breath and bodily sensations to be more present with your suffering.

Working out while distracted enhances your capacity to build grit. If you already exercise without interruptions, take it a step further by incorporating a mantra into your reps, steps, or breaths. Some people are more at ease with phrases like, 'Let go,' or 'Thank you.'

Sit with your emotions

Pause for a couple of seconds the next time you feel lonely, angry, nervous, depressed, terrified, or jealous. Take note whether you were about to pick up your phone to read through Instagram or check your email, or if you were about to switch on the Playstation or grab a beer. Resist the desire and instead sit or lay down (facing down is preferable) and close your eyes. Try to pinpoint a physical sense in your body. Do you have a tight feeling in your chest? In your stomach? Do you have butterflies in your chest? Do you have a sore throat? Do you have a clinched jaw?

Whatever experience you discover, immerse yourself in it completely. Forget about the thoughts that are racing through your mind, and don't try to figure out what emotions you're experiencing if they are hazy. Simply immerse yourself in the physical sensation and feel it thoroughly. For a few minutes, focus on the physical sensation. Then inquire as to what it is attempting to convey to you.

It may appear weird.

However, this is a technique employed in both somatic psychology and ancient yogic practices. You'll be astonished at how much insight you gain from this, and you'll probably avoid the harmful habit of ignoring the feelings you have.

One of the most challenging things we'll ever have to do is sit with our feelings. Some people find it simpler to fight than to feel their emotions. However, the most difficult tasks frequently yield the best results. And this practice will not only enhance your mental toughness but will also improve your relationships, aid in the healing of previous traumas, allow you to break free from unhealthy habits, and propel you to the next stage of personal development.

Name what you feel

It can be difficult to put your sentiments into words at times. It may even be difficult to confess to yourself that you are nervous or unhappy. However, studies show that identifying your feelings reduces their pain. So, check in with yourself a few times a day and ask how you're feeling: set alarms on your phone for the morning, afternoon, and evening.

You will feel better if you can put a name to the mood or combination of emotions. It could be as easy as pausing for a moment to name your feelings to yourself.

Take notes on your phone or on paper with a pen. You can also utilize an emotions word list to help you figure out what you're experiencing. It is critical to connecting with how you feel, otherwise you will be unaware of how your feelings influence your decisions. When you are furious or embarrassed, you may take unnecessary risks.

Take deep breaths

Deep breathing is necessary for developing mental toughness, whether as part of formal meditation or on an as-needed basis. When things get tough, it allows you to better regulate your thoughts, feelings, and, well, breathing. Deep breathing decreases cortisol levels in the brain and body, impairing cognition and helping you decompress.

Hyperventilating might aggravate your symptoms, whereas deep, slow breathing calms you down and lowers your adrenaline and cortisol levels. It allows your stress response to work for you rather than against you, preparing you for constructive action.

Experts recommend two breathing techniques: the 10-second pause, in which you breathe in for 3 seconds and out for 7 seconds, and the box breathing method, in which you breathe in deeply for 4 seconds, hold for 4 seconds and breathe out for 4 seconds. You can also breathe in one nostril and out the other. Deep breathing causes an increase in oxygen flow, which helps reset the deepest areas of your brain and biochemistry.

Talk to someone

There is a significant distinction between "being strong" and "playing rough." Acting tough entails pretending you have no issues. Being strong entails recognizing that you do not have all of the solutions. While it may feel awkward at first, talking to someone might help you develop mental toughness and become a better person.

So, make a real effort to reach out and communicate with your friends and family on a regular basis. A family member or close friend might provide you with a new viewpoint on what you're going through. However, be receptive to professional assistance. Begin by speaking with your doctor to rule out any physical health issues, and then seek a referral to a mental health specialist. Nowadays, you can communicate with a therapist by phone or videocall too.

Exercise gratitude

According to research, appreciative people get various benefits, including increased immunity, better quality sleep, and increased mental strength. Look for ways to be thankful for every day to strengthen your mental muscles. Make it a practice to think about what you appreciate before getting out of bed in the morning or before going to sleep. Finding the silver lining changes how we think about the world, which is an important aspect of developing mental toughness.

Admit your errors

Mentally tough people never try to pretend their mistakes never happened, which is the default posture many take when they realize they've done something wrong. Rather than simply admitting their mistake, many people strive (unsuccessfully) to defend their stance. This just deepens the hole and leads to loss of trust and relationship degradation. Mentally strong people are more open to taking full responsibility for their actions than being proud to admit that they made mistakes. Admitting your mistakes relieves you of your guilt. By refusing to accept you're wrong, you enable the guilt to rot in your stomach.

Admitting your errors also sets a wonderful example for your children. As parents, we frequently feel guilty when we make mistakes in front of our children. But we should not try to hide our flaws or allow shame and guilt to govern us. Rather, we should reframe our missteps as great teaching moments that will better equip our children to negotiate the difficult portions of life. We must be courageous enough to confess when we are wrong, as well as strong enough to correct our error and go on. We must teach our children to be vulnerable, open, and honest, as well as how to transform a mistake into a learning experience.

GRIT-BUILDING HABITS

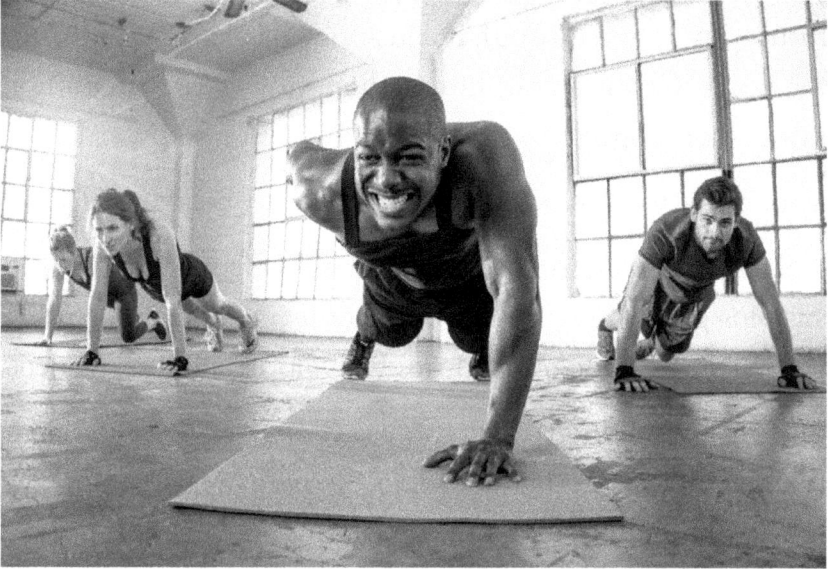

Can you figure out what the most important indicator of success is? You could say it depends on how skilled you are at your craft. Or maybe it's how knowledgeable you are in your field.

No, it isn't.

It's about how psychologically tough you can be when the difficulties keep piling up and the storm lasts a little longer than intended.

It's all about grit.

Throughout our professional careers, one quality stood out as a substantial predictor of success. It wasn't a case of social intelligence. It wasn't good appearance, physical health, or intelligence. It was toughness. On the other hand, Grit is tenacity and a strong desire to attain long-term goals. Grit is characterized by stamina. Grit means sticking with your future day in and day out, not just for a week or a month, but for years. Grit is living life as though it were a marathon rather than a sprint.

Your thinking has the potential to make or break your life.

And mental toughness is the characteristic that fosters and sustains grit. You will build a higher level of grit in your life if you learn how to cultivate and develop mental resilience.

The easiest method to do so is to first establish a clear understanding of what not to do. So, here are some positive habits that will help you develop your mental power, resilience and grit.

I can cite the case of one of my patients who has been following this path for almost two years and now feels much better: more focused, confident and resilient.

Don't be afraid of change

Three years ago, I was in a catastrophic bike accident that left me blacked out on the street and relying on people to come to my aid. And here's the most important thing I learned from it: The only constant in life is change.

You will either have to initiate change or be a victim of it, but you will not be able to avoid it. Your ability to embrace, rather than avoid, change is a sign of mental strength. This does not indicate that you should rush into new projects (I tried, and it wasn't pleasant), but rather that you should be willing to take reasonable chances.

Here's a universal truth: personal development does not occur in our comfort zones. As a result, if you want to grow and expand, you must actively seek change. You must keep moving, try new things, and be willing to push through the discomfort that comes with change.

Recognize that avoiding suffering is more harmful than enduring it. That is the mindset you must adopt if you want to effect the change you desire in your life.

Don't be afraid of solitude; embrace it.

How at ease you are in your skin reflects how well you know yourself. And spending time alone is the only way to understand more about yourself.

After only five days of silence at a retreat in Nepal, I discovered the beauty and calm of stillness and seclusion. Today, I incorporate meditation into my daily routine and make it weekly to spend time alone with my thoughts.

According to research, there are various long-term benefits of isolation. It gives you the ability to accept yourself for who you are. It increases your inventiveness. It boosts your mental health. It also teaches you to accept and love yourself.

People who learn to find comfort alone tend to be happier, less stressed, and have more mental power. And I can vouch for it. So, quit being afraid of isolation. Rather, accept it and create time for it.

Don't dwell on the past

Holding on to the past is nothing more than a form of self-destruction. If you continue to cling to it — if you focus on what you've left behind — you won't be able to see what lies ahead.

Similarly, if you continue to focus on what you don't want, you won't completely invest your energy in what you desire.

The truth is that the past is no longer relevant. What counts now is what you can learn and apply from it. Everything else must be let go of.

Discover how to let go of the past. This frees up your energies to focus on what actually matters: the here and now. Today. At this precise moment. Because what you do right now will shape the next one.

Don't concentrate on your weaknesses

What you pay attention to expands. When I concentrate on my flaws, I accentuate them, and as a result, I feel weak. When I concentrate on my strengths, they become more apparent to me, and as a result, I feel more confident.

According to research, when we focus our efforts on growing our strengths, we grow considerably faster than when we try to address our deficiencies. At work, we grow more confident, creative, and energized.

That is why mentally strong people make it a point to water their strengths regularly. They are aware of their flaws — and acknowledge them — but as long as a flaw does not impede their advancement, there is no incentive to invest time and energy in addressing it.

Don't expect immediate success

The gritty individual treats achievement as a marathon; his or her edge is stamina. And endurance is developed one day at a time.

Athletes do not set world records overnight. Businesses are not created in a single day. Skyscrapers, on the other hand, take years to build. Success does not happen overnight; success is found in the nuances of the process, not in the outcome of the result. You expect immediate results because you overestimate your abilities and underestimate how long true change takes (it's okay, I've been there before).

The magic, however, occurs in the constancy of action rather than the rapidity with which it is carried out. So, if you want to create mental resilience, you should adjust your mentality. Slow down and stay consistent as a habit. Concentrate on your progress and perfect the procedure; you will begin to see the desired outcomes in time.

Don't give up after a setback

A half-year of entrepreneurship took me to realize this: there are no failures, only lessons and experiences. As a result, I've realized that failure is the only route forward.

Failure teaches you what not to do so that you will be in a better position to succeed the next time you attempt. Failure is not a step back from where you want to be; rather, it is a step closer to your goal.

What you consider as a hindrance to your development is actually what propels you forward. And the worst thing you can do after falling is given up and never get back up.

If you wish to improve your mental fortitude, you must totally adopt this viewpoint. Engulf it and wrap it about you like a cloak. Recognize that failure, not an achievement, fosters resilience. Make it a habit to get back up after falling.

Do not contrast yourself with others

The notion that we are in competition with others is a self-created illusion created by our scarcity mindsets. It's one of the most difficult things to cease, but if you're aware of it, you can stop yourself.

Make it a practice to remind yourself regularly that the world is bountiful and that the advancement of someone else's success does not hamper yours - in fact, and it might propel you forward. Seek to learn from others in your fields who have achieved the level of accomplishment to which you aspire.

I now see myself as a modest yet gifted student who regularly works hard to improve his art while also looking up to and learning from the teachers around me.

Success is unique to each individual. Create your own definition of success, as well as an achievement list to measure your progress. This allows you to compare yourself to the prior you.

Don't focus on what you can't change

Mentally powerful people recognize that the only thing they have control over is the present moment and what they do with it. And it is this mindset that feeds grit.

When you pay attention to something you can't control, you suffer from imagination and give up your power. When you direct your attention to what you can control, you deliberate about your attitude and spend your energy.

This practice keeps you upbeat, energized, and motivated. You enter what I refer to as the Sunshine State of Mind quadrant of life.

Avoid making the same mistakes again and again

This was one of my most serious weaknesses. It is all too simple to revert to hazardous recurring behavioral habits. I still do it now and then. But I'm a lot more aware of it now, and I try not to make the same mistake more than twice.

Before brushing yourself off and getting back on that horse, take some time to contemplate and notice why you fell off in the first place before attempting to ride again. Recognize that you made a mistake. Accept it as is. Accept responsibility. Understand what happened and what you can learn from it.

Making the same mistakes over and over is not only an indication of mental weakness; it is also a sign of a lack of self-awareness.

So, if you notice yourself slipping into the cracks, stop and catch yourself in the act. Prevent yourself from entirely engaging in yet another behavioral error by practicing greater self-awareness. You'll be creating a web through which increased mental strength can pass.

Don't indulge in self-pity

Life can be difficult at times. Things may not go exactly as anticipated. For want of a better word, "stuff happens." And, like joy and happiness, melancholy is a natural emotion that we should never avoid. The fact that we linger on our misfortunes, on the other hand, is what destroys us.

When you moan about things 'not being fair' in your world, or think that other people have it 'much better than me,' or even act as if the world is against you and is out to get you because you're so unlucky, you're playing the victim role in an otherwise extremely generous life.

This is not a grit-inducing behavior.

Here's what you should do instead: Allow yourself to fully feel what you are feeling, but keep in mind that your viewpoint has the potential to change your situation. Have the ability to recognize the light that can come from your current situation.

Don't be afraid to act

The cycle of developing self-confidence is as follows: the more you do something, the more competency you gain at it, the more you fuel your inner self-belief, and the more confident you get at it.

Fear equals curiosity.

It is not your responsibility to combat that fear; rather, it is your job to take one baby step in the direction of that dread.

Make it a habit to act because it is action, not thought, that produces clarity and confidence. Become a master of your fears, and, as a result, you will be confident by default. Don't feed your anxieties; instead, feed your faith - and cultivate the resilience to keep going.

Don't be afraid of empathy

Perhaps this habit leans more toward emotional intelligence, but given that the feelings we experience are triggered by the concepts we focus on, we can agree that empathy and compassion are an extension of mental power.

This is something I've been actively working on seeing the world through the eyes of others and realizing that my actions, words, and thoughts affect not only my life but also the lives of those around me.

And, more importantly, it is about being compassionate with yourself because one cannot offer what one does not have.

<u>What Is Important to You?</u>

By incorporating the 12 behaviors listed above into your daily routine, you will be able to create better mental strength. You will learn to accept anything life throws at you because when the storm comes, you will not flee; instead, you will stand solid, face it, and say:

"I'm tough. No, you do not."

NAVY SEAL TRICKS TO TRAIN MENTAL TOUGHNESS

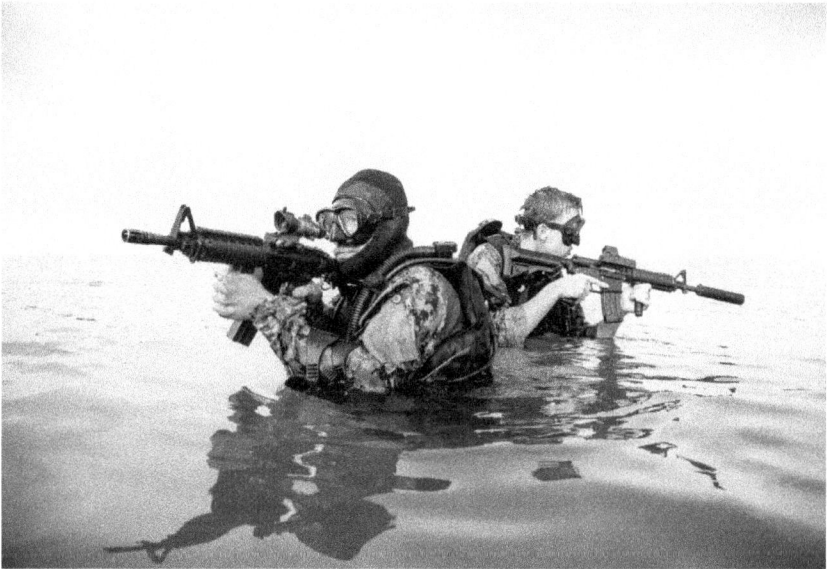

Those who thrive in life have a strong mental toughness.

For those who are unfamiliar, the Navy Seals are the primary special operations force of the United States Navy. It is physically, emotionally, and cognitively demanding work. The majority of those that try out for the Seals do not make it. Mental toughness is what distinguishes successful applicants from those who are sent home.

As it turns out, mental toughness isn't simply necessary for success if you want to be a Navy Seal. Instead, it is critical for everyone. Whatever your aim is, you will need mental toughness to accomplish all of the following:

- Take action on a consistent basis;
- Overcome failures, roadblocks, and setbacks;
- Ignore your detractors; and
- Maintain your motivation even when things get difficult.

The question, therefore, becomes, how can mental toughness be developed? And the answer is through studying the Navy Seals. Here are five Navy Seal mind-tricks to help you psychologically toughen up so you can go to work on your goals and keep going until you reach them.

Increase the stakes

Navy Seal Chad Williams argues that you should boost the ante when working toward a goal to ensure that you persevere until you succeed. That is, consider the following:

"What exactly is at stake?"

The greater the stakes, the more inclined you are to persist. That is, the bigger the stakes, the more mental fortitude you will be able to summon.

Assume your goal is to complete a 10K run. Assume you handed your sister $50 and told her she couldn't give it back to you unless you run a 10K. It's quite likely that you'll give up before you reach your goal.

Why? Because training for a 10K requires a lot of hard work, and $50 is a tiny investment. But what if you tell yourself that the following is at stake:

- I'll shed 25 pounds by training for a 10K. I'll be healthier, I'll be able to move around more easily, and I'll look better.
- If I complete a 10K, I will be providing a terrific example for my children.
- Developing the self-discipline required to run a 10K will help me reach my other objectives.

Now that there's more at stake, you're more inclined to stick with it, right? In reality, Williams deludes himself into feeling that everything is at stake. He tells himself that if he fails to meet his aim, his family will be executed.

Most people, of course, will not want to go that far. You may, however, tell yourself something like this:

- I'll be overweight and sickly for the rest of my life if I don't run the 10K.
- My kids will never respect me again if I don't run the 10K.
- I'll never have the discipline to fulfill any of my other life goals if I don't run the 10K.

It may appear dramatic, but you are more likely to endure until you reach your goal by convincing your mind that there is a lot at stake.

Recover quickly from the unexpected

Several Navy Seals have authored books about their training and how they learned to be psychologically tough in order to endure the life-threatening situations that they are regularly forced into.

I was reading one of these books a while back and came across numerous interesting gems. The book argued that bouncing back swiftly from the unexpected is an important component of mental toughness.

When Navy Seals are getting ready to go on a mission, they are briefed on the situation they will be in. That is, they are informed of their situation and what to expect. For example, if they need to rescue someone from a ship, they will be provided information like this:

- They will be shown the layout of the ship.
- They will be informed of the number of passengers:
- They will be instructed on the weapons that anyone on board may carry.
- They will be shown how to navigate around the ship without being noticed.
- They will be informed of the location of their target: and so on.

However, about 100% of the time, things do not proceed as planned. For example, once on board the ship, the Navy Seals can come upon a wall that isn't intended to be there. At this stage, what does a Navy Seal do? They don't, for example, do the following:

- Stop to consider who is to blame for not anticipating the presence of a wall.

- Stop whining: "Oh, that's usual. They're missing a wall!" or "How are we going to get this done right now?"
- Give up and return

The Navy Seals would almost probably be killed if they did any of these things. As a result, they incorporate the wall into their calculations automatically. They specifically do the following:

- Recognize and accept the presence of a barrier right away.
- Maintain your cool.
- Continue your journey.

If you want to be mentally robust, you must learn to recover swiftly from the unexpected. By saying yourself, "Acknowledge; Accept; Adapt; Act," you can trick your mind into overriding its desire to dispute with what is happening.

The power of visualization

During their training, the Navy Seals are instructed to repeatedly imagine themselves successfully executing any task that is presented to them. They are preparing their minds for what is to come by using imagery. They're winning mentally to win on the battlefield. Whatever goal you're attempting to attain, envision yourself persevering, overcoming difficulties, dismissing critics, and shutting out your inner critic.

If you "see" yourself conquering these obstacles in advance, your mind will not have to determine what to do when encountering them in real life. It will already know how to keep going in any situation since that is what it has been trained to do.

To improve your mental toughness while working toward a goal, train your mind beforehand by envisioning it.

Say a mantra aloud

I recently finished reading Unleash the Warrior Within by former Navy Seal Richard Machowicz (Mack). When Mack was preparing to become a Navy Seal, he received a photograph of a friend's brother who was also a Navy Seal. The photograph shows the friend's brother and several other Navy Seals preparing to skydive out of a plane.

"A man can only be beaten in two ways: if he gives up or if he dies," it said on the back of the photograph. Mack transformed that remark into a mantra: "Not dead, can't quit."

He said this phrase continually throughout the remainder of his training, and he credits it with assisting him in becoming a Navy Seal. After all, being mentally tough is much easier when your mind chatter is conducive to mental toughness.

Adopt the mental chatter of the mentally tough by repeating Mack's phrase or creating your own. Here are several mantras for mental toughness:

- I'll either do it or die trying.
- Only I can get me to quit, and I'm not going to allow myself.
- It is not an option to give up.

Recite your mantra whenever someone attempts to persuade you to quit or when the voice in your head becomes negative. Reciting your mental toughness mantra over and over can trick your brain into thinking that the only option is to keep going.

Concentrate on what is right in front of you

Most of us have lofty ambitions. This could contain objectives such as the following:

- Starting a profitable business;
- Traveling all across the world;
- Completing an Iron Man race, for example.

When a goal is really large, it might be difficult to stay motivated and psychologically tough from the moment you take the first step toward achieving it until you cross the finish line.

Dividing your goal into small chores tricks your mind into continuing when the end line is far away. Then, all you have to do is concentrate on the subject at hand.

For a Navy Seal, this could mean focusing just on running until they reach the bridge a few miles away, then running until they reach the top of the hill, then running until they cross the river, and so on.

It could mean one of the following things to you:

- Writing the next blog post that you will publish;
- Making a 5-minute video for your online course;
- Making five cold calls to potential sales leads; or
- Completing a 10-kilometer bike ride.

Breaking down your huge ambitions into tiny jobs and then focusing on the work in front of you can trick your mind into staying mentally tough. After all, it's difficult to convince your mind that it has to be mentally tough for a year, but you can deceive it into thinking it simply needs to be mentally tough for the next hour.

Stages of mental toughness

One recurring question I've heard over the years of researching high-level special operations fitness is whether I have any recommendations on becoming more mentally strong. I don't want to come out as a grumpy old coach, but *there are no easy tips*!

There is no magic potion that will make mental toughness appear in your life. Mental toughness and resilience are acquired gradually, often over the years, and are frequently achieved through the following stages:

Motivation

In the Navy SEAL culture, it is said that "the motivated find the teams." This is correct, but the motivation must evolve into much more. We all need that initial spark, that reason why you desire to do anything to improve yourself. This is the easiest part because many people are *highly motivated* when they first find a new objective. Motivation can suffer after the work to accomplish this new goal is completed. Motivation is only going to get you started. Maintaining motivation occurs only when the phases listed below are met, which is a time-consuming process. The difficulty here is that time frequently presents stumbling blocks in the form of administrative headaches, physical injuries, or illness. You may feel as if you are beginning from scratch all over again as time passes, but you must keep pushing forward.

Persistence

Webster's Dictionary defines persistence as "the trait that allows someone to continue doing something even when it is difficult or opposed by others."

If inspiration is the first step, persistence is the second. No matter how many rejections you receive along the way, you must persevere. Every day, you must begin moving on the proper path toward your goal. Everything you do should help you get closer to your objective. *Good habits* are formed by continuous perseverance.

Habits

Every one of us is a creature of habit. Habits are daily events that have to be part of the calendar (religiously) so that missing them makes you feel terrible. It is just as difficult, if not more difficult, to break bad habits as it is to form new ones. You frequently have to do both to attain new goals that you are motivated to pursue. After several weeks of working toward your goal, doing the tiny things to help develop your foundation, you will discover that you have formed a habit. Be patient throughout this period, as developing a habit takes time.

Discipline

Without discipline, you will not be able to achieve your goal. Discipline is what gets you moving when you are tired and unmotivated to continue. Discipline necessitates a laser focus on your goal — you must constantly remind yourself that you must get to work doing the things that will improve you, such as learning, exercising, making money, and moving forward. Finding a weakness and turning it into a strength takes perseverance. Similarly, you may require discipline to help you let go of your ego and seek help.

If you don't feel like you have all of the answers and aren't getting anywhere, it may be time to seek help. Discipline is not simply associated with military success; we all require it in everyday life.

So, how can you develop discipline?

Find something that motivates you first, and then enjoy learning more about it. Determine what you must do to reach your goal. Create sub-goals and a timetable. Continue to have fun along the road by doing daily chores that will help you get closer to your goal. These chores could include schoolwork, swimming or running, lifting weights, or anything else requiring continual practice before seeing results. You will have achieved a working level of discipline after you have made this practice a habit. You will soon discover that you are more disciplined in other aspects of your life as well.

Finally, you will have developed mental toughness. You must master the preceding phases before proceeding to the ultimate stage of the process. There will be times when you are physically drained and beat down, and your mental toughness will help you find that second wind, or "the fuel when the tank is empty." This is frequently part of the apex of the challenge that you set for yourself years ago. It will come to this at some point. There is only you and no one else.

How seriously do you want it? I am a firm believer that you cannot measure someone's heart, but you can put it through rigorous testing. Some people believe that you are born with mental toughness, or it is impossible to have it. It's a little of both, in my experience as a coach and as a person. It is possible to develop mental toughness, but it may take years. Many people begin the process with a background in athletics, hard work, challenging life situations, committed study hours, rejecting critics, proving others wrong, and completing difficult projects just through pure work effort that needs you to never quit.

Building a never-say-die work ethic is the final consequence of every challenging feat that requires everything you have. Set a goal, chart a course, stay focused, and *never give up!*

MENTAL TOUGHNESS AND SPORT PERFORMANCE

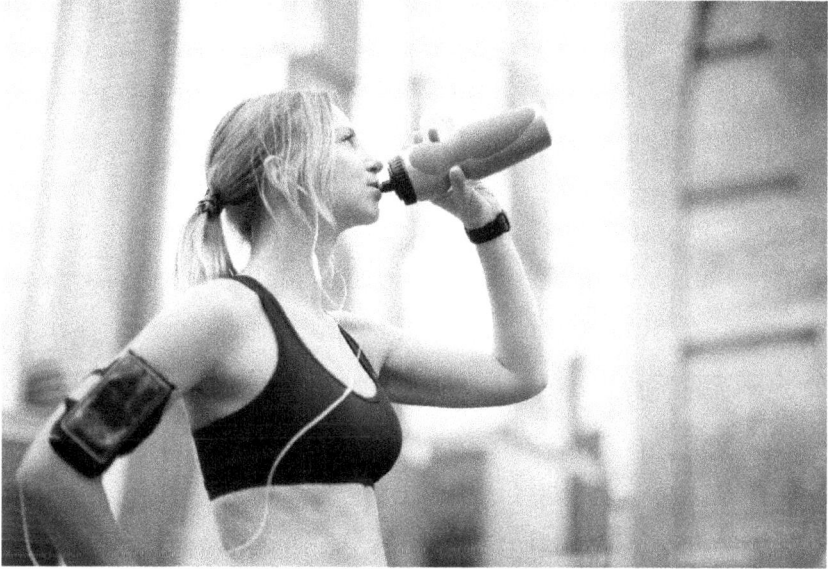

Many athletes seek the solution to becoming "mentally tough," and many athletes are unsure of how to create it. Worse, many athletes and coaches have no idea what mental toughness is or how it might benefit their performance.

People hear elite athletes and Olympians extol the merits of mental toughness training and how mental toughness was the driving force behind their outstanding sports success.

"Football is so much about mental toughness, it's digging deep, it's doing whatever you need to do to help a team win," said Tom Brady, quarterback of the New England Patriots.

Athletes' biggest opponent is a lack of mental toughness. A lack of mental toughness leads to players giving up, giving in, tanking the match, and giving less.

Your level of athletic success is proportional to your level of mental toughness. To be psychologically tough, you must be willing to do what most athletes are not willing to do.

First, let us debunk the myth of mental toughness...

Many sportsmen feel that mental toughness is something you are born with. You either have mental toughness, or you don't, according to the sentiment... You could not succeed in your sport if you were not born with the mental toughness gene.

But this does not have to be the case. You are completely accurate that mental toughness training is required for success, but you are completely incorrect in believing that you cannot become mentally stronger.

Some athletes are more mentally tough than others, such as those who have faced adversity throughout their life and are used to rebounding. I'm thinking about LeBron James and Michael Jordan, just to name a couple of athletes that overcame adversity. And dealing with adversity is part of developing mental toughness. Mental toughness is an attitude, and attitudes are formed solely by you.

You may deconstruct the way you believe about yourself or your potential to succeed if you are the one responsible for your views. By altering your thinking, you will alter your feelings about yourself, which will alter how you act, train, and compete.

Mental toughness is not only an attitude and not something you are born with; it is also a habit.

In sports, mental toughness isn't something you pull out of your back pocket when there are seconds left in a game, or when a 3-foot putt is required to win a tournament, or when you're up to bat with the bases loaded in the ninth inning.

Mental toughness necessitates a steadfast commitment to your sport's problems consistently. You must focus, train, and develop your mental toughness habit on a regular basis.

When mental toughness training becomes a habit, you will be able to perform at the peak of your athletic potential. You are also more prepared to deal with hurdles, interference, and challenging conditions without losing confidence or motivation.

The more you train, the more fit you get in terms of mental toughness. When you quit exercising, your fitness level drops. If you don't take care of your mental fitness regularly, your mental toughness begins to deteriorate.

In other words, mental toughness isn't an all-or-nothing situation. Mental toughness comes in varying degrees. This is fantastic news because mental toughness training can assist all athletes.

You will notice a considerable boost in your performance as your mental toughness reserves rise.

Athletes' mental toughness qualities

Look for a solution, not an excuse

Mentally tough athletes don't make excuses when things don't go their way. Instead of blaming others, they accept responsibility for their actions, return to the drawing board, right the ship, and try again.

Adapt

Instead of doing things the same way every time, mentally strong athletes seek out new ways to challenge themselves, pushing themselves to the limits of their potential. Mentally tough athletes recognize that what they did yesterday has led them to where they are today. However, more work is needed today to get them to where they want to go tomorrow.

Focus their efforts on items that improve performance
Mentally difficult athletes concentrate on things they can control. Mentally tough athletes don't dwell on the past, feel sorry for themselves, or worry about things outside their own control. Mentally strong athletes concentrate on what they can do right now to overcome performance challenges and offer themselves the best chance of success.

View the past as a helpful source of information and nothing more

Mentally tough athletes learn from their own and others' mistakes, then let go of the past and go forward. Mentally tough athletes view the past as mental preparation for future performance. Mistakes, failures, and setbacks do not define mentally strong athletes; rather, they serve to fortify their will.

Take risks

Mentally tough athletes recognize that fear of failure hinders them from fully dedicating themselves to and reaching success in their sport. Athletes with a strong mental fortitude seek out opportunities to push themselves outside of their comfort zone. Mentally tough athletes approach obstacles with excitement rather than dread and anxiety. They refuse to remain ordinary and recognize that they may fall short sometimes, but it is worth taking the risk in order to achieve great things.

Persevere in the face of failure

Mentally robust athletes are never defeated by failure. Mentally tough athletes recognize that failure is only another step on the road to success. Mentally tough athletes believe that failure is not final and never give up on their goals.

Strive for excellence rather than perfection

Mentally tough athletes have a goal in mind, but their emphasis is on the actions necessary to achieve that goal. Athletes with mental toughness recognize that peak performance is a marathon, not a sprint. Each step they take brings them closer to their ultimate aim. They are not humiliated by mistakes, do not strive for perfection, push themselves to the limit, and strive for constant improvement. Mentally tough athletes recognize that they will make mistakes along the way and that these mistakes are both critical turning points on their path to brilliance.

Focus on their talents and abilities

Mentally tough sportsmen do not try to please others or resent the achievement of other athletes. They concentrate on themselves, their talents, improving themselves, putting their game plan into action, and reaching the goals they set for themselves.

Talent might be overrated

There are hundreds of gifted athletes who never reach the pinnacle of their sport. In fact, 75 percent of all young athletes drop out of sports due to a lack of talent, but because they lose interest in sports and lack the mental toughness to compete at higher levels.

Without mental tenacity, talent is useless. When it comes to regular performance, training can be mediocre. However, combining mediocre talent with mental toughness allows good athletes to achieve great things.

Olympic athletes and mental training

During the Pyeongchang Winter Olympics, we witnessed numerous outstanding performances. Mental toughness is a vital component for every athlete to execute a gold medal performance.

Great Olympians have a high level of self-confidence, are able to filter out distractions, manage their arousal level, are goal-oriented, and exhibit a healthy form of perfectionism, according to research published in the Journal of Sports Sciences.

When it comes to sport psychology, mental toughness is one of the most commonly used concepts, yet there is no consensus on defining it.

Researchers G. Jones, S. Hanton, and D. Connaughton defined mental toughness as an athlete's capacity to surpass the competition in managing demands and exhibiting consistency, drive, focus, confidence, and control under duress. They also discovered that mental toughness was both innate and cultivated through time, implying that an athlete who does not appear to be "born with it" can absolutely cultivate it.

Mental toughness is essentially a set of mental talents that include unwavering self-belief, resiliency, motivation, attention, and the capacity to perform under pressure as well as manage physical and emotional discomfort.

Mental skills training is used in sport psychology to help players build mental toughness. Mental skills training include examining players' strengths and shortcomings and developing a program that focuses on key areas important to their sport and their specific needs.

While each athlete's needs will vary, there are some tactics that many Olympians adopt.

Goal-setting

To give a successful performance, Olympians will employ a variety of goal-setting tactics. While they may end up winning a medal or finishing in the top three, they will also set performance and process goals.

Performance goals are self-referential and may include the desire to set a new personal best. Process goals focus athletes' attention on the execution of technical factors required for success. They are the "hows" and "means" of accomplishing a result or performance goal.

For example, a figure skater who wants to win a medal and successfully execute his quad jumps may shift his focus to the aspects within the jump that he knows he can — and must — do to land each jump. This will also boost his confidence and reduce any distracting thoughts of failure or things he has no control over, such as his opponents.

Focusing on the outcome might sometimes distract some athletes and force them to become their own worst enemy.

Self-talk

Self-efficacy is an athlete's unwavering belief that they can overcome a task. It is, without a doubt, the foundation of any great performance. Self-talk is a strategy that can boost self-efficacy and performance.

The mental discourse we have with ourselves is referred to as self-talk. We have over 50,000 thoughts per day. Thoughts are powerful and can have an impact on an athlete's confidence. While athletes can't document all of their thoughts in a given day, they can participate in constructive self-talk. Affirmations of their power and cue words that pump them up or calm them down are examples of such conversation. It can consist of basic reminders of where their focus should be and what they need to do.

Successful Olympians expertly manage their thoughts, ensuring that they are their own best friend at the top of the slope or walking out onto the center ice. Finally, this method has the amazing power to make an athlete feel confident, in control, and prepared to confront any obstacle.

Imagery

Imagery is one of the more difficult abilities to master, but when done correctly, it allows Olympians to visualize themselves performing their discipline from start to finish as if they were doing it in real-time.

Imagery entails envisioning the real activity that an athlete wishes to perform while engaging all of their senses. What's more, when it's thoroughly practiced, the muscles involved in the action in the real-life fire in the same order and rate – as if the activity were actually being performed.

Many notable Olympic athletes spend hours imagining what they want to do and how it should feel in preparation for competition. They would even play out worst-case scenarios, feeling the strain and discomfort, and rehearse their right response. When it comes time to compete, they are prepared for any situation. It is undoubtedly the most difficult aspect of their preparation, but they must perform well when it matters the most.

We see athletes practicing imagery the most in sliding events like luge and bobsleigh. The gravitational force that these athletes are subjected to endangers their health and inhibits their capacity to physically practice their sport.

Arousal management

Olympians have a sweet spot for how they want to feel when they are performing at their peak. This is their optimum degree of arousal. Some athletes love to be hyped up, while others prefer to be so quiet that you wonder whether they are aware they are about to compete.

Like a thermostat that controls the temperature of a house, successful Olympians have their degree of arousal dialed in.

If they discover that they have strayed beyond this zone, they will restrict it.

An athlete, for example, can reduce arousal by taking deep breaths from their diaphragm and engaging in self-talk to become more relaxed. Similarly, an athlete might increase their arousal level by taking shorter breaths or listening to music. The most crucial thing here is that the athlete feels in control of their emotions.

When it comes to peak performance, being mentally tough undoubtedly gives any athlete an advantage over their opponent. While certain athletes may have this intrinsic ability, it can surely be harnessed and improved.

Successful Olympians understand the value of mental toughness. Most world-class athletes recognize that training on their mental talents is just as vital as working on their physical and technical abilities.

Debunking myths about mental toughness

One of the most often questions I get from coaches is, "How can I make my athletes more psychologically tough?" Despite how popular the term "mental toughness" has become, the concept remains a mystery. In this piece, I'll open that box and debunk four damaging beliefs about mental toughness. Coaches must dispel these stereotypes to assist young athletes in developing mental strength and supporting their overall mental well-being. However, before we get there, we must analyze our existing situation. That is, why are coaches concerned about developing mental toughness in today's youth athletes?

Today's youth generation is, for lack of a better word, mushy. It's not always their fault. They are growing up in a different environment. Everyone receives a participation award. Kids are simply less willing to work hard, to persevere in the face of failure, and to grind it out. And parents are not allowing their children to fail. Parents prepare the way for their children in the classroom and on the court. 'Helicopter parents' who used to hover have evolved into 'snowplow' or 'lawnmower parents,' pushing all obstacles out of the way so that children never have the opportunity to learn how to deal with pressure and failure.

I work with some parents who, like this coach, use the snowplow on occasion. I also work with calm and loving parents. Consider that, like players and coaches, parents do not exist in a vacuum. Parents' pressure when navigating the youth sports system (the privatized one with a hefty price tag and one year-round training option) is difficult. We must approach these difficulties with a focus on contribution rather than blame. Coaches must collaborate with parents, players, and administrators to ensure that every youth athlete has a positive sporting experience.

So, how can we teach young people to grow in the face of hardship in sports? To begin, we must refute some generally held fallacies regarding mental toughness in sport (and life).

Myth #1: Mentally difficult athletes always have positive thoughts/emotions

More positivity does not imply greater mental toughness. Mental toughness includes both apparent and imperceptible acts such as thoughts and emotions. People who exhibit mental strength, on the other hand, may not always think self-affirming ideas or feel completely assured. Being too optimistic and unrealistic in our thinking can undermine our performance and motivation; when we establish unreasonable success expectations and consistently fall short, we are less willing to work hard and persevere through problems. Mental strength, on the other hand, necessitates realistic views about our talents. Regardless of the situation, it necessitates trusting and focusing on our individual process — on improving rather than proving oneself.

Mentally strong people are also conscious of "bad" ideas and feelings. They flourish in both positive and bad settings, which can be both external (e.g., game conditions) and internal (e.g., fearing failure). Athletes with mental toughness dare to accept and analyze unpleasant thoughts/emotions in order to get insight into their circumstances. For example, suppose a player is irritated due to a team dispute. In that case, that athlete demonstrates mental toughness by addressing their "what" (emotion) and "why" (reasons for the feeling) rather than hiding their dissatisfaction (which likely makes team dynamics worse).

Mentally tough people do not ignore negativity. To move forward and behave following their ideals, they accept all aspects of their experience (e.g., use team conflict to strengthen group relationships).

Myth #2: Mentally tough athletes are neither emotionally nor psychologically sensitive

This misconception stems from Tom Hanks' memorable comment in *A League of Our Own*, "There's no crying in baseball!" Being mentally tough does not imply that you have fewer emotions or are less sensitive to them. Mentally powerful people, as debunked in Myth #1, are acutely aware of their emotions. We must be willing to identify and validate our emotional experiences to be mentally strong. In doing so, we acknowledge that emotions are a normal part of being human: we are not alone in experiencing grief, shame, and fear, and we are not wrong for doing so. Mentally strong athletes can then select how to effectively progress toward achieving their goals by mindfully digesting their emotions. That is, individuals can evaluate why they feel the way they do and whether those emotions assist or hinder them in achieving their goals.

Myth #3: Mentally tough people are willing to endure more (physical) hardship

The amount of wind sprints an athlete can complete is NOT a measure of mental toughness. I believe, or hope, that coaches are moving away from jogging young athletes till they puke as a manner of developing mental toughness. This antiquated approach is not only ignorant but also irresponsible. I am not implying that all fitness training is harmful. However, incorrectly training athletes and putting their physical/psychological health in danger while claiming to be a "developing character" is abusive.

Athletes with high mental fortitude exercise hard and smartly. Hard and smart training entails guiding athletes to push their physical limitations in developmentally appropriate ways while simultaneously establishing boundaries to promote long-term performance, development, and well-being. Mentally tough athletes recognize that adequate rest and recovery are essential components of their training regimen. They are consistent, disciplined, and patient. And they have the humility and bravery to leave the game if they are hurt when "simply playing through it" for short-term glory jeopardizes their long-term aspirations.

Myth #4: People who are dealing with mental health concerns are mentally weak

Mental health difficulties are becoming more frequent and noticeable at all levels of competitive athletics. Professional athletes' advocacy efforts (e.g., Kevin Love and Michael Phelps) have contributed to initiate an open discussion about mental health issues. These efforts are critical since mainstream sports culture promotes a "no pain, no gain" ethos and discourages discussion of mental health. Given the rise in mental health concerns among Generation Z athletes (and kids in general), it is vital to talk about mental health and dispel the myth that mental health struggles and toughness are mutually exclusive.

Mental strength is comprised of (acquired) characteristics and talents that enable individuals to thrive in high-performance conditions. Everyone can enhance their mental strength, but the procedure varies from person to person. While athletes with mental health disorders may face more adversity, this does not imply that they are mentally inferior. In truth, athletes display and gain amazing mental power as a result of, rather than as a result of, their mental health difficulties, as Michael Phelps claimed in certain interviews.

Tips for building mentally strong athletes

Coaches are in an excellent position to dispel myths regarding mental toughness to assist youth players in developing mental toughness and changing sport culture. Here are four practical suggestions to help you get started.

<u>Work with parents rather than around them</u>

We may work alongside parents rather than around them if we communicate our approach and set boundaries ahead of time. We must explain our "what" (philosophy), "why" (rationale), and "how" (methodology) (boundaries that are necessary for us to coach effectively). When coaches accomplish this, we provide a framework for parents to get involved in consistent ways to support their child athlete's growth process. Encourage parents to let their children fail in conversations. More importantly, communicate to parents and players that failure is essential for learning and progress. Failure as required feedback communicates that "success" is about committing to a young athlete's individual process — to being the best version of oneself and growing better every day — rather than the end (i.e., winning).

Create a "brave" space in training and games for athletes

Coaches develop brave spaces by putting athletes in (ideally) demanding situations that push them to their "learning" limits. Coaches must recognize and reward instances when players have the fortitude to take chances and attempt difficult tasks in order for athletes to learn to accept physical and mental difficulties and uncertainty. We need to tell athletes that these are ideal opportunities for improvement so that they recognize the value of pushing themselves outside of their comfort zone.

Boundaries exist in brave spaces, and coaches must assist players in establishing them. Athletes must be taught how to work out smartly and listen to their bodies. Along with encouraging athletes to push themselves, we must emphasize that rest is a component, not an absence, of training.

Encourage athletes to become more conscious of their emotions and thoughts

Encourage athletes to regard their internal experiences, whether positive or negative, as normal and potentially valuable in reaching their goals. Assist athletes in defining their ideals and long-term objectives. Check in with players regularly and provide reflective questions to assist them in exploring why they feel or think the way they do and whether or not those feelings or thoughts are helping or hurting them reach their goals. Instead of repressing or avoiding perspective-taking, assist them in becoming aware of and receptive to their own (and others') emotions.

Use social media to assist athletes in developing mental toughness

Social media has an impact on how our young people see failure and how they acquire mental strength. Social media is frequently utilized to make ourselves appear perfect. We rarely see (or upload) photographs of failure or difficulty, preferring to see championship celebrations and college signing day images.

While I don't want to discourage individuals from celebrating their accomplishments, coaches may assist players in understanding that social media focuses on the "good" aspects of others' processes.

As coaches, we can utilize instances of professional athletes overcoming adversity to initiate discussions with youth athletes. We may also look critically at what we share (and encourage athletes to do so) by asking ourselves, "Is my post an attempt to prove myself (and appear perfect) or document my process?"

Improve your mental toughness while running

Running is one of the most popular and widely practiced sports on the planet. In 2017, about 60 million people in the United States alone participated in running, jogging, and trail running. In 2017, more than 110 million people walked for fitness in the United States. One of the primary incentives for Americans to begin running or jogging is to improve their fitness. In 2017, approximately 24% of Americans reported that exercise was the primary reason they began running. Weight worries and the desire to compete are two other prominent reasons why Americans take up the sport. Almost 80% of American runners continue to run to be healthy or in shape. Relieving stress and having fun are two of the main reasons why individuals in the United States continue to run as a sport.

How mentally tough are you as a runner? We talked about seven crucial characteristics that define a champion's mentality. Resilience, focus, strength, preparation, vision, openness, and trust are some of these features.

The good news is that mental toughness does not have to be innate. Everyday running activities might help you develop mental toughness. Anyone who aspires to be a better runner can cultivate the qualities that create a mentally strong runner.

Each of us begins at a different physical and mental starting place. We all have strengths on which to build. You have the best chance of attaining your running goals if you develop these abilities and practice them on a regular basis.

Now that you've identified the characteristics of psychologically tough runners, how do you translate these characteristics into helpful actions that will improve the way you train and race? Use these five suggestions to help you develop your mental toughness as a runner.

Build your performing edge toughness attitude

Because the mind and body are so inextricably linked, having the right toughness attitude is essential for success. First, the proper internal state must be formed. A fantastic performance can happen simply and smoothly when you feel good on the inside. The right mental state can bridge the gap between what you think you can do and what you really do. It can mean the difference between simply having the talent and reaching your full potential.

Develop a mentally tough outlook

Peak performance is made possible by positive energy. Concentrate your attention on what is conceivable, on what can happen, on success. If you want to be a psychologically tough runner, instead of moaning about the weather or criticizing the competitors, focus on what you can control:

your thoughts, emotions, training form, and how you perceive each scenario. You have a say in what you think about yourself.

Visualize mental toughness on a daily basis

Spend 10 to 15 minutes each day mentally rehearsing your goals. Through deep abdominal breathing, put yourself in a relaxed state. Then, as vividly as possible, imagine what you want to achieve in your jogging. You can recreate one of your best mentally demanding performances in the past. Then channel all of your positive sentiments of self-assurance, vitality, and strength into your mental preparation for an approaching event. Visualize yourself doing it correctly. Finally, continue to use your imagery during the event.

Establish a relaxed focus

Work on keeping your concentration for extended periods to become more mentally robust. You can tune in to what is important to your performance while tuning out what isn't. You can simply overcome distractions and regain control of your attention. As you concentrate more on the immediate task at hand (your stride form, how you feel, etc.), there will be less place for negative thoughts to enter your head. You'll be psychologically tough in any situation.

Use strong words to increase mental toughness

To prepare psychologically for your next event, try repeating the following phrases:

- *Whatever it happens, I stay positive and mentally tough*
- *I fully enjoy every part of my workout*
- *I project confidence and enthusiasm*
- *I am both mentally focused and physically relaxed*
- *Going fast feels effortless*
- *I am in my element; I am totally immersed in my running*
- *I am tuned into what I am doing each moment*
- *I am a powerful, mentally strong runner*

MENTAL TOUGHNESS IN THE WORKPLACE

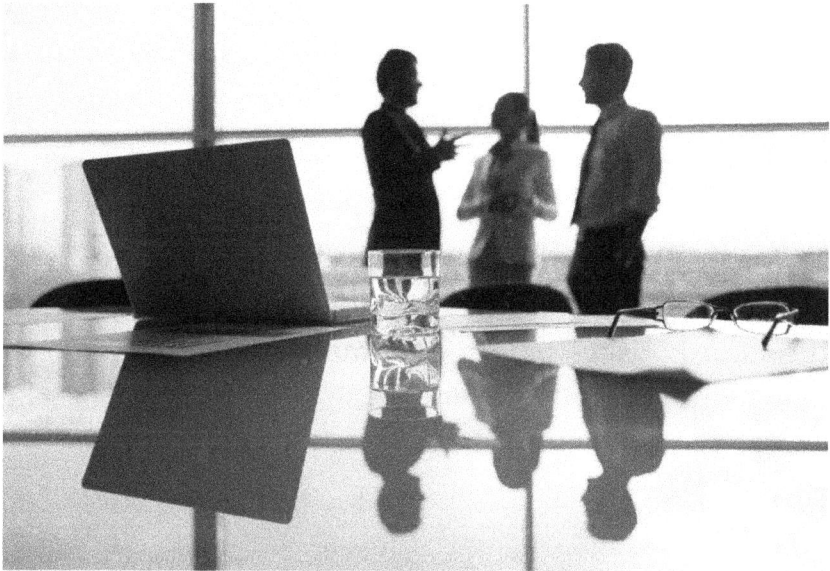

Every employee has been subjected to work-related stress at some point in their career. After all, any work (regardless of how much you enjoy it) can cause stress. So, how can we cope with work-related stress? Mental toughness may be able to assist us in dealing with this.

Mental toughness entails being able to manage under strain while maintaining self-belief and focus. However, mental toughness demands intensive training and preparation to be effective due to the length of working practices (e.g., the frequency of the day and the length of the working year). Implementing specialized mental abilities is one factor that can improve mental toughness.

Process goals

Goals are a frequent method that we use to keep our motivation and desire to reach targets high. The capacity to define and meet process goals can only help to boost confidence and self-belief. Too frequently, as performers, we set goals that do not take into account the result. For example, we could set a goal of completing a specific task. This aim is ineffective since we are struggling to satisfy standards that might harm performance and mindset. As a result, creating process and performance targets should be considered. Using our first example, we may decide to impose a time limit in order to finish the assignment. For example, I will finish this assignment in five days. Furthermore, the task can be broken down into basic processes, allowing for the achievement of shorter goals. Shorter goals promote a positive mindset and allow us to sustain the inner drive to reach our overall outcome goal.

Positive self-talk

There is no doubt that working conditions are demanding and stressful. As a result, we may experience a variety of emotions and thoughts that occupy the mind. Positive self-talk can assist in supporting and facilitate this process. Negative thinking is replaced by positive self-talk. For example, "I'm in pain and worried that I wouldn't be able to finish this assignment" might be substituted with "I intend to do this assignment within the time range I've established." Positive self-talk allows neuronal pathways in the brain to function more positively than negative thinking. Indeed, negative thinking affects neural circuits, which confuse the brain and contribute to worry, hindering performance. Consider your mental space. You can have a mind-space that is clouded with hurdles and impediments or a mind-space that is clean of clouds and filled with sunlight.

Resilience

Because of the nature of working practices and their demand, resilience is essential for performance. Resilient workers can deal with hardship and have a strong desire to complete assignments. Knowing what to accomplish and how to pace work demands is what resilience entails. Resilient workers have the psychological capacity to deal with the physical and mental challenges of their jobs.

Working methods have undervalued the use of mental toughness. On the other hand, companies should be encouraged to undertake mental toughness training to support their staff. Such training has the ability to not only assist people with job responsibilities but also to strengthen their thinking and enhance their well-being.

Things to consider about self-awareness

Mentally tough employees are the foundation of a mentally tough team. Insights about ourselves in terms of work-related habits increase our mental prowess and allow for candid self-awareness in the workplace. Understanding your inherent traits—how you react, respond, and relate—

can help you achieve your goals. By becoming self-aware, you are more likely to discover your strengths as well as your limitations, allowing you to work on each of them to become more successful at work and in life.

Natural characteristics, strengths, and talents

There are a variety of tests available to determine your inherent abilities and talents. Some experts use the following formula to calculate a person's strengths: Talent multiplied by investment equals strength. Your natural recurrent patterns of thought, feeling, or action are referred to as talents. They are the innate, natural abilities that you can use productively. Another alternative is the KOLBE evaluation, which analyzes instinctive strengths and helps you discover what comes easily to you.

Many large corporations use these technologies and other unique approaches to assist them in hiring, mentoring, and ensuring that their employees are in the correct seats. Their employee-owners are committed to discovering and utilizing their abilities within their teams and among their peers. Learning their own capabilities as well as being aware of the strengths of others allows them to operate better as a team.

Developed habit

Learned behaviors are those that you are born with but do not know how to do. These are taught behaviors, either by trial and error or by observing others. Aside from the nurturing, we receive at home, and we are frequently influenced by the people we associate with.

How frequently did you hear this as a kid? These influences can be both positive and negative, emphasizing the importance of self-awareness, particularly in the workplace. Seeking out leaders to serve as mentors can be beneficial in ensuring that any newly learned behaviors help you grow and advance in your role.

Workplace environment

It is critical to work in an environment that makes you feel at ease, safe, motivated, and joyful. When assessing yourself and your current employment, you should have a firm grasp of how you feel at work. Always look for a company that values its employees and where executives seek to create a culture that people can be proud of. If you're not pleased with work, you're not going to be happy at home, right?

Learning from one's flaws

We've all got them. We all have flaws that cause us to stumble and fail. It is difficult to learn from failure, to learn from our mistakes, and, simply, to accept our flaws! Accepting our flaws, on the other hand, can be freeing. When you acknowledge them, you become aware; you may become the finest version of yourself when you are aware.

<u>Having the finest work-life balance possible</u>

According to revisesociology.com, the average American spends approximately 1842 hours each year at work, equating to 50% of your total awake hours in any given working day. Why would anyone want to be unhappy at work when we spend half of our time doing so? It is critical to living the greatest work-life balance!

How to develop mental toughness at work

To state the obvious, today's workplace is stressful. The digital shift is fueling a culture of isolation and distraction. The pace of labor is quickening. And the ability to stay continually connected to the office gives us the impression that we are never offline.

Many of the problems we confront at work are caused by factors outside our control. You can't always do anything about a difficult boss or coworker, an unreasonable task, increased external competition, strange office dynamics, or a constantly changing environment. But there is one thing you can always control: yourself. This includes your attitude, worldview, explaining style, and adaptive capacity. While each of these characteristics is significant on its own, when they are combined, they become extremely potent.

Fortunately, mental toughness is not a fixed or innate trait. It may be nourished, grown, and enhanced by our decisions and the perspectives we embrace both in and out of the office. Here are some strategies for developing the kind of mental reserves that can let us deal with anything that today's job can throw at us.

Positive thinking equals positive outcomes

Believing in your ability to succeed is the first step toward success. Learning to maintain your positive in the face of adversity is a great measure of mental strength. When you face negative people who don't believe in you or make a mistake, it might be difficult to remain to believe in yourself. Don't let naysayers influence your thinking. Maintain an optimistic attitude and believe that if you persevere, you will eventually triumph.

Maintain consistency

The ability to continually work toward accomplishment is an important aspect of mental toughness. Mentally strong people tend to be very constant, sticking to their goals even when they feel less driven or receive disappointing results. Develop your mental fortitude by regularly putting in the effort: go to every practice, put in the hours, do the research, and keep showing up!

Create new habits

Developing new habits will assist you in achieving consistency and increasing your ability to persevere through difficult moments to achieve success! It usually takes 2 to 3 months for a new habit to become routine. Taking pauses, speaking with coworkers, setting monthly (or even weekly and daily!) goals, writing those goals down, and other professional routines can aid with mental toughness and focus. Consider which habits will help you succeed, and then begin adopting them into your daily routine.

Make no excuses

Mentally tough people do not offer excuses; instead, they move ahead even when difficulties come. That is not to say that there aren't instances when we face significant difficulties. Life can be difficult, and this can have an impact on your ability to concentrate! Take care of yourself, resolve any issues that arise, and then, rather than using setbacks as an excuse to abandon your goals, recommit to them and keep moving in the direction of your aspirations.

Concentrate on yourself

Judging your success in comparison to the success of others can be very discouraging. Concentrate on what you've accomplished and what you hope to do in the future. Be so focused on your own goals that you can't be distracted by envy or jealously over what others are doing.

Avoid thinking in terms of all or nothing

If you only allow for black and white, all-or-nothing, success or failure, you will miss out on everything in between! This way of thinking might be defeatist because you may feel as though you should abandon the entire effort if you make one mistake. Instead, mentally resilient people can perceive mistakes as opportunities to learn.

Determine what motivates you

What is your driving force? Are you pursuing a goal because you are enthusiastic about it, or are you attempting to impress your boss? Internal motivation is a characteristic shared by mentally difficult individuals. This is because when we are sincerely devoted to our final goal, we are more eager to put in the effort required to achieve it. It is critical to feel motivated at work, so spend some time to figure out what motivates you. It could be that you want to help your coworkers, that you want your product or service to be the best it can be for your customers, or that you want to learn new things. Knowing what inspires you allows you to tap into that enthusiasm and continue working hard toward your goals.

Don't try to do it alone

Trying to succeed on your own may appear to be a sign of strength, but it will not benefit you in the long run. Even Olympians competing in solo sports have teammates, coaches, and an entire support system behind them! Having the accountability of others might help you consistently show up and work toward your goals. In the context of your workplace, it can be beneficial to bring in mentors to assist you if you become stuck. Coworkers are designed to be your teammates, and they can often assist you with skillsets you lack or cheer you on when you need them.

Utilize your inherent abilities

Know your strengths and weaknesses — they're both crucial! While you can develop at anything if you put in the effort, it's also a good idea to concentrate on what you're naturally excellent at. When you enjoy what you do and believe you are good at it, it is frequently simpler to be enthusiastic about your work.

Develop self-confidence

Continue to show up and make an effort to prove your ability to yourself over and over. This means that if you claim you'll finish a project by the end of the week, you put in the effort and meet your deadline. Or, if you say you'll start a new habit, you commit to making time for it. The more you keep your promises to yourself, the more you will have faith in your mental power.

Make use of your blunders to your advantage

Allow setbacks to not be the end of the path. Complications, difficulties, and even failure are all part of the trip. Mitigate the damage as much as possible, figure out how to prevent those same issues next time, gain whatever lessons you can, and then keep moving toward your goals! Allow challenges to be a source of progress rather than a reason to give up.

Have a good time and enjoy the process!

When you care about the work you're doing, perseverance is easy to cultivate. Put your time into initiatives that interest you, surround yourself with coworkers you care about, work for a firm whose goal you support, or find another way to feel enthused about your work!

The mentally strong employee

Companies all have one thing in common: they want to be successful. They can't do it with mediocre employees. Employees who are easily distracted or sidetracked will not benefit the organization. Companies can profit from recruiting tenacious staff. People with grit know how to deal with failures and disappointments and persevere in the face of adversity.

Perseverance gives people the determination to think beyond the box and overcome challenges. A leader can choose to instill grit in their team to achieve greater success. Teaching grit can give your team a boost and keep them anchored in the face of adversity.

This tenacity may be taught in a variety of ways with the appropriate approach and effective leadership. One strategy for incorporating mental toughness into your culture is to expose your staff to inspiring resources and inspirational articles to learn how to overcome obstacles. As a leader, you can also try to understand your employees' points of view to become more understanding and use their experiences as a learning opportunity.

Coaching / Mentoring

Having a mentor who can offer support and encouragement is an important part of endurance. Having someone to help you is a great approach to motivate your employees to perform more successfully and efficiently. While a mentor should not promote employees whose work is subpar, he or she should take the time to make suggestions for improvement and constructive comments.

Another wonderful idea is to get instruction and development from someone who is an expert in a certain field. In this situation, the consultant would assist in the mentoring of staff on mental toughness. This therapy could involve classes on overcoming difficult obstacles and achieving goals despite the stress and strain that comes with attempting to perform at a high level. A mentor can offer employee counseling and advice on development, which can be a great motivator.

Create Self-Sufficiency

A leader must instill trust in his or her employees. Self-government is the first step toward mental toughness. It is critical to developing the skill to regulate yourself while no one else is present. Inform your employees that you have faith in them. You recruited them for a purpose, and you know they can accomplish the job. This boosts confidence tremendously. Self-reliance defines a person's genuine character and how strong they are.

Cultivate perseverance

Everyone picks what kind of day they want to have in the morning. It is time to demonstrate mental fortitude. Hold a focus group and present a problem that has to be solved to your staff. It will begin to put mental fortitude to the test, and it will benefit the team's cohesiveness. Having people operate as a collaborative unit, whether they like each other or not, is part of practicing perseverance. Communication from a corporate leader to an employee is critical in keeping a strong mentality and assisting people in performing at the maximum level.

Recognize the role of grit

A leader who wants their personnel to show grit should start by discussing grit. Explain how persistence can help you achieve your goals. Discuss tales in which people persevered and obtained what they desired. You might also use this time to share your own tales of persistence that have led you to where you are today. Spiega il significato degli obiettivi e come la pratica contribuisce al successo. It sometimes stimulates folks to hear instances of what you require from them.

One's attitude defines grit. It is about seeking, striving, discovering, and never giving up. Great leaders understand how to persuade their staff to work towards a common objective. Employees sincerely feel that if they persevere, they will be able to achieve their goals. Employees that are self-assured and psychologically resilient will help the company flourish no matter what problems arise.

MENTAL TOUGHNESS AND PARENTING

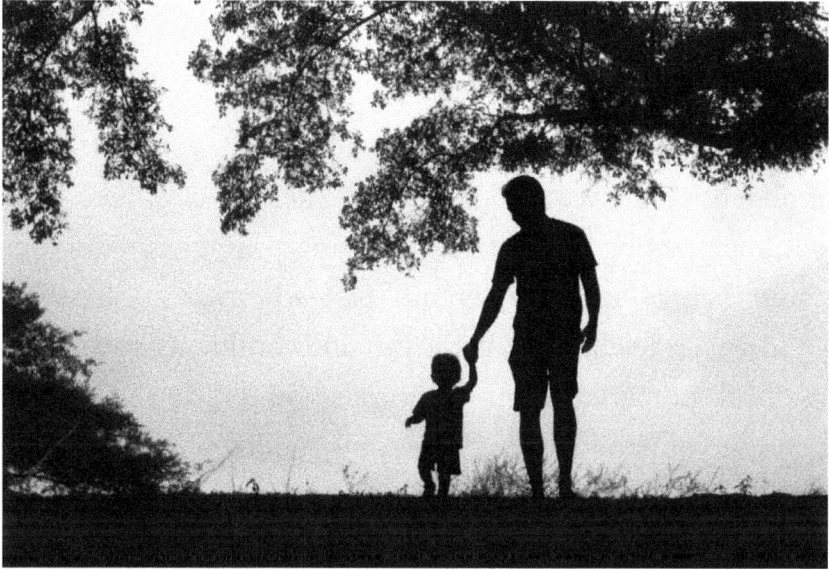

Mental toughness does not imply being tough on the outside. It is about having the inner courage to continue and pursue personal objectives. It's about being comfortable in your own skin. It is about having the courage to step outside of your comfort zone to progress.

It is about identifying possibilities rather than threats and approaching pressure, stress, and problems with a positive attitude. Mental toughness stems from professional sport, where it has been employed successfully for over 30 years, but it also applies to everyday life - for both children and adults.

According to research, mentally robust children perform up to 25% higher in tests. They sleep better, pay more attention in class, and have bigger expectations. They also make a smoother transition from junior to secondary school, report less bullying, and are less prone to engage in anti-social behavior.

Mentally strong children are better prepared to face the problems of the world. To be clear, mental toughness does not imply acting tough or suppressing feelings. It's also not about being cruel or defiant. Instead, mentally healthy children are resilient, with the grit and confidence to achieve their full potential. There are things you can do as a parent to assist your children in developing mental power.

Teach kids how to be mentally tough

Psychologically strong children can deal with issues, recover from failure, and manage adversity. A three-pronged approach is required to assist children in developing mental strength. There are three approaches to assisting children in developing mental fortitude.

- Assist them in learning to regulate their emotions so that their emotions do not control them.
- Demonstrate how to take positive action
- Teach them to substitute more realistic thoughts for negative ones.

There are numerous parenting practices, disciplining approaches, and instructional materials available to assist children in developing mental muscle. Adapt your strategy to your child's individual needs.

Show children how to be tough

One of the most effective ways to teach children mental strength is to model these skills in your own life. Children learn how to respond to various situations by observing their parents. So, try to be aware of your mental toughness and focus on areas where you can improve. Here are some ideas for teaching your children how to be mentally strong.

Mental strength as a role model

The best method to assist your child in building mental strength is to show them how to be mentally strong. Discuss your own goals with your child and demonstrate that you are taking steps to get stronger. Make self-improvement and mental strength a priority in your own life, and avoid the behaviors that mentally strong parents do not engage in.

Show your kids how to overcome fears

If your child avoids anything frightening, he or she will never learn the confidence needed to deal with discomfort. Whether your child is afraid of the dark or meeting new people, help them conquer their concerns one small step at a time. Cheer them on, praise their achievements, and reward them for being courageous, and they'll realize they're a capable child who can handle moving outside their comfort zone.

<u>Mental toughness can be taught</u>

Look for ways to provide your children the tools they need to be psychologically robust. Working with kids in various settings allows you to instill the mental toughness required to deal with uncomfortable emotions and handle difficult situations. Here are some particular ways you may teach your children to be psychologically strong in the face of adversity.

Teach specific skills

Discipline should be about teaching your children to do better the next time, not punishing them for their errors. Use consequences to teach specific abilities like problem-solving, impulse control, and self-discipline. These abilities will assist your child in learning to act productively even when confronted with temptation, difficult situations, and terrible setbacks.

Teach emotional regulation techniques

Don't try to console your child when they're upset or cheer them up whenever they're down. Instead, teach them how to deal with unpleasant feelings independently, so they don't become reliant on you to keep their moods in check. Children who understand their emotions and know how to manage them are better prepared to face obstacles.

Allow your child to make mistakes

Teach your child that making errors is part of the learning process so that they do not feel ashamed or embarrassed if they make a mistake. Allow for natural consequences when it is safe to do so, and discuss ways to prevent making the same mistake again.

Develop tough abilities

Building mental power in children also necessitates paying attention to their confidence, independence, and self-esteem. Work with your children to fine-tune these aspects of their lives while encouraging healthy practices that strengthen their mental fortitude. Here are some ideas for expanding on what they've learned about mental toughness.

Encourage positive self-talk

It's difficult for kids to feel mentally strong when they're constantly putting themselves down or forecasting disasters. Teach your youngster how to reframe negative beliefs for them to think more realistically. The best way to assist children in overcoming adversity and performing at their best is to develop a realistic yet optimistic viewpoint.

Forge character

Children require a strong moral compass to help them make sound decisions. Make an effort to impart your values to your child. Make time for life lessons that reinforce your principles regularly. Instead of winning at all costs, highlight the value of honesty and compassion.

Children who understand their beliefs are more likely to make healthy decisions, even if others disagree with them.

Let your child experience discomfort

Although it may be tempting to assist a child when they are in distress, doing so will reaffirm to them that they are helpless. Allow your child to make mistakes, allow them to be bored, and insist on responsibility even when they don't want to be. Struggles, with support and instruction, can help your child develop mental strength.

Prioritize gratitude

Gratitude is an excellent antidote to self-pity and other negative behaviors that can inhibit your child from developing mental strength. Assist your child in affirming everything good in the world so that they will recognize that they have plenty to be glad for even on their worst days. Gratitude can improve your child's attitude and promote proactive problem-solving.

Assume personal accountability

Accepting personal responsibility is necessary for developing mental strength. When your child makes a mistake or misbehaves, allow for explanations but not excuses. If your child attempts to blame others for how they think, feel, or behave, correct them.

What mentally strong parents don't do

Raising mentally strong children who are prepared to face real-world issues necessitates parents abandoning unhealthy — yet popular — parenting approaches that deprive children of mental strength.

Of course, it is not easy to assist children in developing mental muscles; it requires parents to be mentally strong as well. It's difficult to watch children struggle, force them to face their anxieties, and hold responsibility for their mistakes. However, these are the kinds of experiences that children require to develop their full potential.

Parents who prepare their children's minds for a life of meaning, happiness, and achievement avoid the following common mistakes:

<u>They do not support the victim mentality</u>

Your child is not a victim because he or she was cut from the soccer squad or failed a class. Life is full of rejection, failure, and unfairness. Rather than allowing their children to throw pity parties or dramatize their misfortune, mentally strong parents encourage their children to transform their difficulties into strengths. They assist people in identifying methods in which they can take constructive action regardless of their circumstances.

They do not parent out of a sense of guilt

Guilt can lead to various bad parenting behaviors, such as giving in to your child after you've said no or overindulging your child around the holidays. Mentally strong parents understand that, while guilt is unpleasant, it is bearable. They refuse to let their sentiments of guilt stand in the way of making sound decisions.

They do not position their child as the center of the universe

It's easy to let your life revolve around your child. Children who believe they are the center of the universe, on the other hand, grow up to be self-absorbed and entitled. Mentally strong parents teach their children to focus on what they have to offer the world rather than what they are entitled to.

They do not let fear dictate their decisions

Keeping your child in a safe bubble could save you a lot of stress. However, keeping children overly safe inhibits their development. Mentally strong parents see themselves as guides rather than protectors. They let their children go out into the world and experience life, even if it is frightening to let go.

They do not give their children authority over them

Kids with too much power decide what the family will eat for dinner or plan how they will spend their weekends. Growing up to be more like an equal — or even the boss —

isn't good for youngsters. Parents that are mentally strong empower their children to make proper choices while maintaining a clear hierarchy.

They do not expect perfection

Expecting high standards from children is healthy, but expecting too much from them will backfire. Mentally strong parents understand that their children will not excel at everything they try. Rather than pushing their children to be better than everyone else, they concentrate on assisting them in becoming the best versions of themselves.

They do not allow their child to avoid taking responsibility

A psychologically healthy parent will not say things like, "I don't want to burden my children with duties." Children should be allowed to be children." They anticipate that children will pitch in and gain the skills required to become responsible citizens. They actively encourage their children to accept responsibility for their actions and assign them age-appropriate responsibilities.

They do not protect their child from pain

It's difficult to watch children suffer from hurt feelings or anxiousness. Tolerating discomfort, however, requires skill and firsthand experience in children. Mentally strong parents offer their children the support and assistance they require in dealing with pain, allowing their children to acquire confidence in their capacity to deal with whatever challenges life throws their way.

They do not believe they are responsible for their child's emotional well-being

It can be tempting to comfort your children when they are unhappy or to soothe them when they are angry. Regulating your children's emotions, on the other hand, inhibits them from developing social and emotional abilities. Mentally strong parents teach their children to be accountable for their own emotions and not rely on others to do it.

They do not keep their child from making mistakes

Whether your youngster gets a few questions wrong on his math assignment or forgets to pack his soccer cleats for practice, mistakes can be the best teachers in life. Mentally strong parents enable their children to make mistakes and face the inevitable repercussions of their behavior.

They don't mix up discipline and punishment

Punishment entails making children suffer as a result of their transgression. Discipline is the process of teaching them how to perform better in the future. While mentally strong parents do impose punishments, their ultimate goal is to teach their children the self-discipline they will need to make better decisions in the future.

They do not avoid discomfort by taking shortcuts

It is quick and easy to give in when a youngster whines or does your children's tasks for them. However, these shortcuts teach children harmful behaviors. Tolerating discomfort and avoiding those tempting shortcuts requires mental fortitude.

They never lose sight of their values

It's easy to get caught up in the day-to-day business of homework, chores, and sports practices in today's fast-paced environment. Many individuals lose sight of what is truly essential in life due to their hectic schedules and the pressure to look like the best parent of the year on social media. Mentally strong parents are aware of their ideals and ensure that their family lives in accordance with them.

Sports parents and mental toughness

Sports, whether you like it or not, come with pressure. There will come a day when your young athlete will be given the ball with the clock winding down or will be called upon with the bases loaded. When this occurs, mental toughness frequently determines whether or not they will succeed.

Even if you can't be on the field or court with your young athlete during these circumstances, there is a lot you can do ahead of time to help. Here are five approaches to help you get started.

Refer to your young athlete as a competitor

"Here comes Johnny, our star goalie," or "There goes our little winner." What words do you use to introduce and describe your child?

Use caution when choosing descriptions that highlight only a portion of their identity. They are not always the victors, and they are not always the losers. A father of a friend's athlete once described her as "beautiful little Sara." That's a lot to live up to.

Your children are only athletes on occasion. They can, however, compete in all they do. They are capable of competing in academics, paying attention, and participating in sports. In order to compete, you must first compete against yourself, not against anyone else.

Admire your partner

I find it easier to be a good parent than a good partner. I can love my children, but I also need to love with the assistance of my wife. I have to listen, reflect, emphasize, budget, discipline, strategize, and co-parent with my wife. It requires more effort.

The most crucial relationships take place within our four walls. Our interactions, displays of affection, and disagreements with our spouse or partner reflect how our children will perceive the outer world. Also, keep in mind that children see everything. It is important how you act. Remember, you have the authority to establish what your children consider to be "normal" conduct. They will approach others in the same way if they detect aggressiveness and hatred towards one another.

Consider ownership rather than buy-in

There is a significant distinction between ownership and buy-in. Ownership is more powerful because your children want to play. Buy-in implies that participating in sports is the idea of someone else — usually yours. Isn't it true that the best parenting happens when your children believe they came up with the idea?

Competitors who take charge of their game will take ownership of the team. Before each season, clarify your position and ask your children for comments. Allow them to pack their bags, arrange extra practices, and make use of their leisure time. After the initial talk, do not intervene unless their safety or health is jeopardized.

Avoid sending text messages or emails

Unfortunately, we rely far too heavily on texting to communicate. It is appropriate for short messages and reminders but not for complex matters, especially when emotions are involved. It's not so much what you say as it is what they hear.

The majority of coach-athlete and parent-athlete issues stem from a communication breakdown. We text essential messages to our children far too often instead of setting up a time to discuss.

Overcoming adversity helps children build mental resilience. They must be able to successfully interact with their coaches and teammates. However, if they are not allowed to use their voices, they will be unable to speak up when necessary.

Do not discuss other players, coaches, or teams

Sports are all about winning, but they're also about losing and improving. Nobody enjoys losing, but it isn't fatal. We assist our children to develop mental fortitude by exposing them to disappointments and hardship.

But all too frequently, we try to improve it. We provide an escape, an excuse if we try to erase their ownership by blaming someone else. If there is an escape route, they will take it and learn how to use it. Bad decisions, bad plays, and poor execution occur, but what lessons are we imparting when we say, "It wasn't your fault; it was something else's"? According to such thinking, it must be due to something else when our children perform well and win. We can't have our cake and eat it too.

Final tips for fostering your kids' mental toughness

Every parent wishes the best for their children. As parents, we understand that life will throw many curve balls at our children. We want children to be resilient, but we also want them to be able to do more than just deal with setbacks.

We want them to live their lives to the fullest. To guarantee that children thrive, we must encourage them to be interested, proactive, positive, and self-assured in their talents and interactions. We require mental toughness from them. How can you assist your children in developing mental toughness?

Tip #1 - Challenge

Challenge your children and help them see obstacles as opportunities to learn. Tell them it's okay to fail and that you've failed many times. Remind them that every failure has taught them something. Encourage your child to 'try something new.

Tip #2 - Confidence

Assist your children in developing self-belief and becoming confident in their interactions. Inform them that it is acceptable to feel terrified or have fears in the classroom. Accepting and embracing these feelings is the first step toward overcoming them. Remind them of the strength of YET! If they say they are unable to accomplish something. Tell them they can't do it YET! Remind your children that everyone has a mind and thoughts of their own. It is healthy to form your own opinions, and it is acceptable to differ from time to time.

Tip #3 - Commitment

Teach kids how to set and achieve goals. Set simple goals with your children, such as brushing their teeth, making lunch, or packing their school bag. Praise your child's efforts rather than their results. Remind them that it's okay if they don't get it perfect the first time; every skill takes practice and time to master.

Tip #4 - Control

Teach your children about self-esteem, help them feel comfortable in their own skin, and help them control their emotions. Inquire with your child about what went well at school today. Find three positives and investigate why they were pleasant experiences. Discuss setbacks, such as being passed up for a role in a play, losing a game, or being unable to do something. Remind them that setbacks are a normal part of life and that they will have another chance. Discuss the incidents that they disliked during the day and how they reacted to them. Explain how kids can choose how to react to these experiences to empower them.

CONCLUSION

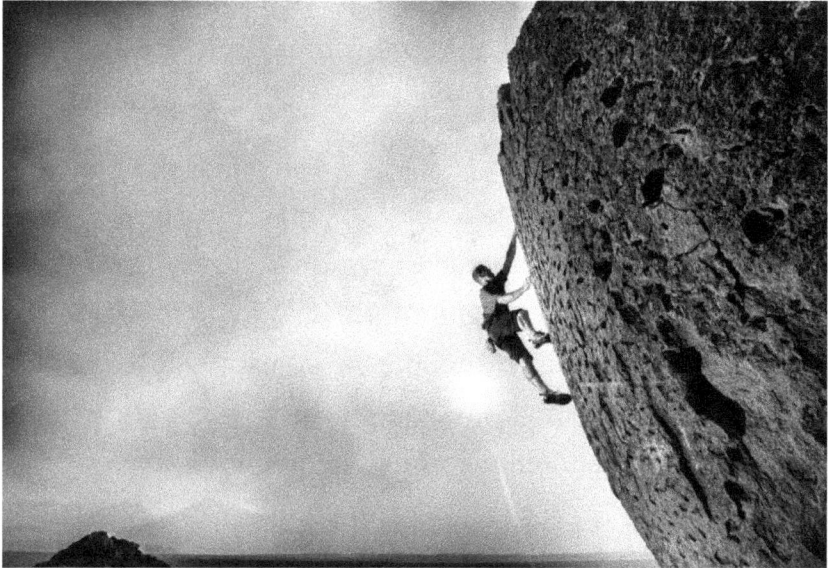

Mental toughness is a combination of resilience, the desire to learn and progress, interpersonal confidence, and belief in one's talents.

Mental toughness is closely related to traits like tenacity, resilience, and grit, but it is a larger notion. Many people define resilience as the ability to rebound from setbacks. Resilience, by definition, is reactive. Mental toughness complements resilience by adding proactive characteristics such as seeking a challenge, change, and opportunity with self-assurance.

The distinction between the two is commonly stated as follows: *"resilience makes you survive, mental toughness makes you thrive."*

Winning, being macho, being insensitive, or being self-centered are not characteristics of mental toughness. It is about being self-aware and comfortable in your skin. There is fortitude and inner strength in refusing to give up and believing that you can win even though the odds are stacked against you.

Mental toughness is a malleable personality attribute, which means it can be cultivated. Developing mental toughness usually involves training you to deal with stress more successfully by making fundamental adjustments to the way you think about situations and teaching you the methods and strategies that mentally tough people utilize.

In the pages of this book, I have described several effective mental toughness practices to you in detail. For some, the report and self-help guide are enough to get them started. Some people may require a coaching talk to fully comprehend the outcomes before committing to a course of action.

In any case, don't put it off any longer and start learning about your mental toughness right away!

UP

URANUS
PUBLISHING

www.ingramcontent.com/pod-product-compliance
Lightning Source LLC
Chambersburg PA
CBHW050728030426
42336CB00012B/1464